DYNAMIC ASPECTS OF HOST-PARASITE RELATIONSHIPS

DYNAMIC ASPECTS OF HOST-PARASITE RELATIONSHIPS

Volume I

Edited by

AVIVAH ZUCKERMAN, PH.D.

Professor of Parasitology, Hebrew University–Hadassah Medical School,
Jerusalem, Israel

and

DAVID W. WEISS, PH.D.

Professor of Immunology, Hebrew University–Hadassah Medical School,
Jerusalem, Israel

Academic Press   New York / London

A Subsidiary of Harcourt Brace Jovanovich, Publishers

Academic Press, Inc.
111 Fifth Avenue
New York, N. Y. 10003

Distributed in the United Kingdom by
ACADEMIC PRESS, INC. (LONDON) LTD.
24/28 Oval Road, London NW1

Printed in the United States of America

CONTENTS

PREFACE AND INTRODUCTION

Interest in the study of host-parasite relationships has declined sharply with the development of effective antibiotic and chemotherapeutic treatment of microbial diseases, and during the past 20 years the student of general biology and even of microbiology has had decreasing academic opportunities to gain insight into this area. This has been an unfortunate deficiency, because the study of the interactions of potential hosts and potential parasites remains one of the most interesting and important, aspects of the natural sciences. It is indeed doubtful whether investigations of host-parasite interrelationships are less pertinent today from the perspective of human health, or less rewarding in terms of scientific curiosity, than they were before the introduction of the sulfa drugs and penicillin.

The pathological consequences of contact with parasitic organisms remain a major medical problem in all societies, and the major problem in many. Even where infectious diseases have been brought under relative control today, the appearance and establishment of resistant populations of pathogens and of vectors, and the apparently limited number of specific agents which are available to combat them, have made it clear that there are no short cuts to permanent defense against microbial invaders. We have been afforded more a breathing space than an all-time magic arsenal by the discovery of specific antimicrobial agents, and a growing understanding of the dynamic interplay between potential hosts and potential parasites remains requisite to our continued ability to direct these equilibria in favor of the species we wish to protect.

This consideration becomes even more apparent if we take into account that the relative respite from infectious diseases which some societies have won is based very largely on the erection of artificial bulwarks against the microbial world, and not on any basic changes in the distribution of potential pathogens or in the inherent susceptibility of potential hosts. These barriers are exceedingly fragile. They are entirely dependent on the essentially normal functioning of complex societal and technical structures, and they disappear when these structures become disassembled by natural catastrophe, war or other major social upheavals—to which this century is no stranger. In such circumstances, species once artificially

[VII]

protected, and having had little opportunity of maintaining intrinsic resistance by means of natural selection or acquired immunity, may find themselves critically defenseless. Moreover, these barriers appear diaphanous when viewed in the light of all the possibilities of the appearance of new pathogens and of new susceptibility traits in potential host populations.

The needs for basic, strategic approaches to the maintenance of a constant shield against the world of potential parasites are further underlined if we include within the category of host-parasite relationships the confrontation between vertebrate organisms and the neoplastic variants which arise within them, as indeed we must if we are to view neoplasia as a biological phenomenon (1, 2).

As a subject of fundamental scientific interest, the area of host-parasite relationships has come to be even more important with the rapid accumulation of information on the molecular bases of biological phenomena. The knowledge gained in the past 30 years on the chemical and physical processes which underlie and explain the structure and function of cells, tissues and organisms remains truncated, without a parallel development of understanding of the interaction of these biological compartments with each other. As models for the study of the ecology and sociology of cells and of individuals, the interrelationships of potential hosts and parasites today offer in many instances the technically most feasible and conceptually most attractive possibilities, and no approach to the study of the phylogeny of species or the ontogeny of individuals can ignore host-parasite biology. It goes without saying that this field remains as pertinent today as it was in the past to the student of the cultural and economic history of human communities.

A series of monographs on the "Dynamic Aspects of Host-Parasite Relationships" is timely for still another reason. As special terminologies develop rapidly within each subspecialty of biology, the loss of contact between disciplines and the fragmentation of basic, unifying concepts become increasingly dangerous. An ongoing series of studies on host-parasite interactions, covering the broadest spectrum of models, may help to retain the lines of communication and understanding between the disciplines of biology by emphasizing common principles, while at the same time clearly delimiting those areas in which real biological differences exist.

The term "host-parasite relationship" correctly designates an intimate interaction, or stage of interaction, between two or more distinct organisms.

in which the one benefits while causing damage to the other(s). It is often difficult, however, to assign the term with precision. Partners in biological relationships not infrequently change roles, as the association proceeds, with regard to the benefit or damage which accrues to each one, and gain and loss are elusive and not absolute qualities. A given relationship may be beneficial to one partner in one environmental context, and damaging in another. What is good for the individual organism may, in the long run, be harmful to the species, and the converse is a no less common occurrence. The observer may judge the quality of a relationship at one level of organization and ignore an entirely different quality, perhaps more determinative of the future of the organism, at another. A bacterium causes a severe but limited inflammatory lesion, and its animal host suffers objective symptoms of illness. Some time later, the host succeeds in expelling the bacterial parasite. The host is left with significantly heightened resistance to other, more dangerous microorganisms in his immediate environment, and is perhaps even enabled more rapidly and decisively to defeat an already existing, threatening infection established at another point in his tissues. The species of the host has gained by the experience, in that the survival of the individual may contribute to the phylogenetic process of selection of more resistant members, and in that the heightened acquired resistance of the individual may reduce reservoirs of infection for the species. The species of parasite may also have benefited despite the destruction of individual bacteria, in that a necessary, though temporary, ecological niche may have been found, from which dissemination of some survivors occurred. Clearly, even in such a simplified relationship, the assignment of benefit and damage is a complicated and at least partly relative matter, and the objective observer may even be somewhat uneasy as to whom the epithet "parasite" most properly designates.

The criteria of smaller size and inferior evolutionary status on which the designation "parasite" is often based are not always adequate, as illustrated, for example, by the parasitism of Bdellovibrio on other bacteria not generally more complex, and themselves parasitic on many higher organisms. Moreover, the smaller size and lesser complexity of an organism do not, as such, determine all the interrelated consequences to itself and to the partner with which it interacts.

The appropriate definition of host, parasite and parasitism is even more difficult when viewed from the perspective of the origin of the organisms which play the respective roles at a given moment. It is today considered not unlikely that some of the complex organelles of the cells of higher organisms may represent the ultimate, reciprocally beneficial and now obligatory, symbiotic stage of relationships which may have begun long ago as classic endoparasitism. Conversely, at least some parasitic microbial agents may have originated as components of higher cells which acquired morphologic distinctiveness from the parent cell, although remaining metabolically dependent on it. In the case of neoplastic cells, their immediate derivation from normal host tissue and their frequently close similarity to it have made for a reluctance to classify them as parasites, whereas, on the other hand, their essentially distinct and at least partially independent nature, and the dynamics of their pathogenic interaction with the animal in which they originate, force us so to view them.

It is essential, therefore, that the student of host-parasite relationships maintain a constant awareness of the fluid, changing nature of the phenomena he studies, and of the inadequacy of the usual terminology to define the biological realities before him.

The difficulty of pinpointing the complex, continuous and evolving interactions of living organisms by a set terminology, which is inherently static and thus artificial, is even more obvious in the cases of words like "symbiosis," "mutualism" and "commensalism." These are used today very differently by different investigators, frequently leading to considerable imprecision and even to contradiction of meaning. Accordingly, an attempt will be made in this and succeeding volumes to standardize these terms, along the lines suggested by Henry (3).

"Symbiosis" will be used in the broadest sense of the term to designate all relationships between two distinct organisms which are intimate and of sufficient duration to have an effect on the physiological behavior of one or both. This use of the word is similar to the one originally advanced by De Bary, except that the demand is not made that the two partners must of necessity be of different species. In stressing a sufficient duration of interaction to allow for physiological response to each other's presence, the definition excludes very fleeting contact, of no consequence to the interactants. It is emphasized, however, that symbiotic relationships can span the spectrum of associations from those which not only last for the lifetime of the individuals but may permanently involve the species, to those which may run a full course in a matter of hours or even less, but which nonetheless profoundly affect one or both participants.

"Mutualism" will describe symbiotic associations, or periods in such associations, which are reciprocally advantageous, that is, in which the benefits accrued to each partner appear to outweigh any detriment. "Commensalism" will be applied to those symbiotic associations in which there *appears* to be neither advantage nor disadvantage to either of the participants, and to associations in which only one partner *appears* to profit and the other neither gains nor suffers disadvantage. It is doubtful, however, whether such commensal relationships in fact exist. They imply mutual or one-sided neutrality, and the better all the facets and implications of a symbiotic relationship are understood, the more such areas of supposed indifference shrink. Absolute neutrality in the interplay between organisms appears not to exist in nature, or to be very rare, and assignment of the term commensalism more often than not only states lack of insight into the dynamics of an association.

The idea for this and the succeeding volumes grew out of an advanced seminar on dynamic aspects of host-parasite relationships, consisting of 8 to 10 lecture-discussion periods, which is sponsored annually by the Institute of Microbiology, Hebrew University–Hadassah Medical School, Jerusalem. This course is primarily directed at graduate students in biology and advanced students of medicine, but is also intended to keep faculty colleagues up to date as to new developments in host-parasite studies, and to provide a forum for the exchange of concepts and information. Guests from other institutions in Israel and from abroad occasionally participate as lecturers. Some of the lecturers have been invited to prepare their talks for subsequent publication in these volumes, which thus contain many, though not all, of the seminars given.

The seminars focus on host-parasite relationships as unique biological entities. The determinant role of environment in the realization of the genetic potentials of organisms is analyzed in the light of the special circumstances of their interaction as actual hosts and parasites. Emphasis is placed on the recognition that a given genetic or environmental factor may have very different implications for the normal growth and reproductive capacity of an organism, and for its ability to mount virulence or resistance mechanisms. The stress of the course is thus on the special biology of the interplay among host, parasite and, where this applies, vector, and not on the intrinsic morphologic and physiologic qualities of each.

In each yearly course, the attempt is made to include contributions from divergent areas of host-parasite relationship studies, and to select examples of host-parasite interactions at the organismal, cellular and molecular levels. The topics vary widely, and largely reflect the major scholarly and research interests of the contributors. Subjects marked by a rapid accumulation of new information or of extensive current interest may be represented repeatedly in these seminars and accompanying volumes, to advance and discuss new data and different aspects of the topic, and to allow for varying points of view. Although no attempt is made to offer a systematic or comprehensive survey of host-parasite relationships, it is hoped that over a number of years these volumes will encompass a sufficiently wide range of the facets of parasitic relationships to constitute an ongoing analysis of their basic elements and of their meaning to general biology and medicine.

The contributors to the course may choose to demonstrate original experimental findings, to review critically an area of work or to discuss theoretical aspects of the field in greater depth; and these volumes will, correspondingly, include such different types of communication. In all the presentations, an attempt will be made to provide a sufficiently broad and basic introduction to each topic to orientate those seminar participants and readers who lack intimate familiarity with the background or technical details of a particular subject, so that each problem can then be discussed without sacrificing a true depiction of its complexities, difficulties and ramified significance. By also introducing descriptions of experimental design and new data in the seminars and published essays, it is hoped that the student and reader not yet intimately familiar with the nature of investigations in the area of host-parasite relationships will become more aware of the special approaches, difficulties and challenges which characterize this field.

Jerusalem, 1 Elul 5731   DAVID W. WEISS
(22 August 1971)   AVIVAH ZUCKERMAN

REFERENCES

1. WEISS DW. Immunologic parameters of host-tumor relationships: Spontaneous mammary neoplasia of the inbred mouse as a model. *Cancer Res* **29**: 2368, 1969.
2. WEISS DW (Ed). "Immunological parameters of host-tumor relationships." New York, Academic Press, 1971.
3. HENRY SM. Foreword, in "Symbiosis." New York, Academic Press, 1966.

BDELLOVIBRIO BACTERIOVORUS AS A MODEL FOR THE STUDY OF BACTERIAL ENDOPARASITISM

MOSHE SHILO

Department of Microbiological Chemistry,
Hebrew University–Hadassah Medical School, Jerusalem, Israel

INTRODUCTION

Host-dependent (HD) bacteria, which live within the cells of other organisms, are widespread in nature and many cases of such intracellular habitation have been described, involving both mutualistic and parasitic associations.

Absolute endoparasites are microorganisms which have lost certain independent vital functions for which their host compensates at its expense. Thus, among the parasitic protozoa, certain trypanosomes, especially the bloodstream forms of the *T. vivax, T. congolense* and *T. brucei* groups, no longer possess the cytochrome type of terminal respiration. Having no oxidizable reserve, these forms must depend for respiration and motility on host substrates (1). Among intracellular parasite bacteria, members of the Chlamydiae group, which cause trachoma, lymphogranuloma and psittacosis, are considered to be energy parasites, having lost their capacity to generate high energy compounds (2). Similarly, certain rickettsiae have been demonstrated *in vitro* to depend on an external supply of NADP and ATP.

In endosymbiotic mutualism, on the other hand, vital functions of the host organism are fulfilled or supported by the invading microorganisms, which, in turn, benefit from the association. Certain hosts have developed specific organs, called mycetomes, which harbor microorganisms. These are the rule in animal groups specializing in a single, limited type of nutrition (e.g., blood or sap-sucking insects and wood-eating insects) (3). A kind of intimate endomutualism has been postulated in a cryptomonad lacking chloroplasts (*Cyanophora paradoxa* Korschikoff) containing "cyanelles" which fulfill the plastid function, transforming the host into a

[1]

functional photoautotroph. These cyanelles appear to be endosymbiotic *Anacystis*-like blue-green algae devoid of the typical blue-green algal cell wall containing peptidoglycan. Another example is the ameba *Pelomyxa palustris* which lacks mitochondria, and in which intracellular bacteria seem to replace mitochondrial function under aerobic conditions (5).

The most extreme case of intracellular endosymbiosis may be the postulated prokaryotic origin of mitochondria and plastid organelles of eukaryotic cells. The individuality and semiautonomous growth and division of these organelles, their unique base composition and nucleic acid configurations, their extranuclear division and even mating ability as demonstrated in yeast mitochondria and their double membrane boundaries all argue that they were originally prokaryotes which invaded primitive eukaryotic cells and stabilized as permanent obligatory symbiotic elements within them in the course of evolution (6).

The study of prokaryotic endoparasites might thus provide interesting new insights into the evolution of the eukaryotic cell and its organelles. On the practical side, an understanding of the nature of the endoparasite's dependence on the host cell may lead to the development of rational therapy and, conversely, to biological control of host organisms where these become pests in nature.

In all cases of endoparasitism, the interactions between the host and the parasitic microorganisms are extremely complex. Obligate intracellular parasitism, characterized by intimate spatial and physiological association of the parasite with the host cell, requires a series of integrated mechanisms, each essential for the success of the process. These mechanisms must insure that the parasite locate on and attach to the specific host cell, penetrate into certain intracellular compartments of the host cell, damage host-cell membranes to allow leakage of nutrients into the area where the parasite is developing and, finally, that parasite progeny be released after completion of their developmental cycle.

In general, information on these mechanisms is limited, and a great deal remains to be learned about these processes and of the evolution of endoparasitic states. This paucity of information is due, in great part, to the fact that most endoparasitic systems are very difficult to study experimentally. The growth of endoparasites is host-dependent and often cannot be achieved in defined media. Experimentation with multicellular hosts is complicated by the difficulty of obtaining synchronous infections in whole organs or organisms. Furthermore, *in vitro* studies with tissue cultures of host cells are hampered by their long generation time.

It is obvious that an endoparasitic system in which both host and parasite are bacteria would greatly reduce these experimental difficulties. A system dealing with hosts with short generation times would allow for synchronous infection and would ensure physiological uniformity of the host. Such a system must, of course, have the basic attributes and properties of a typical endoparasitic system: a) the bacterial parasite must have active means to reach its host, to attach to it and to penetrate into a suitable intracellular compartment; b) the parasite must show specificity, i.e., be capable of "recognizing" a suitable host; c) the host-parasite interaction should not result in the gross disruption or lysis of the infected cell before the developmental cycle of the parasitic bacteria is ensured; and d) swarming out and spread of the parasite progeny to new host cells must occur upon termination of the parasite's life cycle.

These criteria appear to be fulfilled in endoparasitic associations involving parasites of the *Bdellovibrio bacteriovorus* group discovered several years ago (7). This group of predatory bacteria attack, penetrate into and develop within the periplasm of other bacteria. Found ubiquitously in soil, sewage (oxidation ponds), and marine and freshwater environments, the known *Bdellovibrio* strains are specifically parasitic on gram-negative microorganisms. The developmental cycle of *Bdellovibrio*, which can be followed in the host and in cell-free systems, terminates in division and in the release of infective progeny. In its intimate dependence on specific bacterial hosts, its active attack and penetration of the host cell, and its complex life cycle in the host's periplasmic space, *Bdellovibrio* offers an excellent model system for studying endoparasitism and the nature of host-dependence at the molecular level (8).

The analogy between *Bdellovibrio* and members of the Chlamydiae is striking. When members of the psittacosis group invade a host cell, the internal architecture of the parasite changes, but it does not lose its morphological integrity at any time during the production of new generations.

Infective particles of *C. trachomatis* and *C. psittaci* are engulfed by suitable host cells and develop, grow and subdivide by fission within phagocytic vacuoles surrounded by the cytoplasmic membrane of the host cell. Multiplication of the parasites involves a complex growth cycle in which large developmental forms, known as the initial bodies, form within characteristic cytoplasmic inclusions. The intracellular growth of Chlamydiae and *Bdellovibrio*, alike, thus takes place in an exocellular space separated from the host cell cytoplasm by the host membrane systems.

Morphological aspects. In their free, motile stage *Bdellovibrio* are usually seen as small rods or vibrios, 2 μm long and 0.3 μm wide. Their size and shape may, however, vary with the strain and with growth conditions. At the anterior pole, invariably the site of attachment to the host, there are rigid, spikelike fibers arising from ring structures built into the cell wall (9). The opposite pole of the *Bdellovibrio* cell bears a thick flagellum of uniform diameter, sheathed along its entire length.

The morphological changes occurring during the sequence of interaction between bdellovibrios and their hosts may easily be followed and timed with the phase-contrast microscope. When host and parasite come together in suitable liquid media, the interaction begins with the violent collision of the anterior pole of the motile *Bdellovibrio* with the usually much larger host organism. On impact, the motile host is usually immediately immobilized, while the attached *Bdellovibrio* shows a rotary motion.

Ultramicroscopic studies of the succeeding stages of penetration have been made by many investigators. Burnham and colleagues (10) made a three-dimensional reconstruction of the process, based on serial sections of ultramicrographs. According to their observations, the first step in penetration following *Bdellovibrio* attachment involves the bulging out of the host's cell wall and membrane at the point of attachment. The parasite then appears to push against the weakened center of the bulge and breaks through the host's outer wall which has slightly separated from the cytoplasmic membrane. The invader thus squeezes into the cell periplasm through the pore pierced in the cell wall, constricting along its length as it penetrates. Ten to 20 min pass between the time of attachment and complete penetration, but the process of actual penetration is accomplished within seconds. After entering the host, the parasite's flagellum is lost.

Recently, Abram and Chou (11) proposed a different penetration mechanism. They suggest that the *Bdellovibrio* must attach to the host cytoplasmic membrane so as to be pulled into the periplasm passively by the contraction of the protoplast and its retraction from the inner cell-wall boundary. This suggestion is based on electron microscopic observations of *Bdellovibrio* attachment to the host cytoplast during and after entry, and upon the experimental finding that penetration does not occur in plasmolyzed, old and washed cells where the cytoplasmic membrane is not compressed against the cell wall.

At the early stage of *Bdellovibrio* growth in the host periplasm, the cytoplasm of the host cell appears to remain intact. However, constant leakage of necessary nutrients and metabolites from the host cytoplasm can be inferred from the regular course of infection when both host and parasite are suspended in buffer solutions. All the nutrients must therefore be supplied by the host (12).

In later stages, the host protoplast decreases in size and finally completely disintegrates. Meanwhile, the *Bdellovibrio* increases many times in size, growing into a long coil which ultimately completely fills the host-cell space. Several constrictions form simultaneously in the *Bdellovibrio* coil. The coil divides into a chain of cells, and this, in turn, separates into individual progeny units. Daughter cells can form even before constriction is completed (13), and move actively within the empty host cell.

When they swarm out of the host-cell ghost, the small, extremely motile and active progeny are immediately capable of reattacking other hosts.

Physiological aspects. Special methods had to be developed for the quantitative study of the physiological requirements and kinetics of the different developmental stages of *Bdellovibrio.*

Attachment is measured by separating free *Bdellovibrio* cells from the larger host cells by a single differential filtration through membrane filters of 1.2 μm mean pore size. With this method, more than 95% of the free bdellovibrios and less than 3% of the host cells pass into the filtrate. By mixing radiolabeled bdellovibrios with an excess of nonlabeled host organisms, the kinetics of attachment can be followed by determining the radioactivity retained on the filters.

Bdellovibrios which have attached to the host but not yet penetrated can be detached by mechanical shearing using a microblender. The extent of active penetration can then be measured by differential filtration. Only bdellovibrios which have penetrated the hosts will be retained on the filter, while free and detached parasites pass into the filtrate (14).

Intracellular growth on synchronously infected host populations is measured by the increase in plaque-forming units on lawns of the host (15). Other bacteriophage techniques, such as one-step growth experiments and single cell bursts, are also applicable in the measurement of the intracellular development of bdellovibrios (15, 16).

Recognition of and attachment to the host are primary requirements for successful parasitism. Even in chance encounters, the active motion and directional movement imposed by the polar flagellum assure a high probability of contact at the attachment pole. Observations of motility show a definite correlation to attachment. Chelating agents, organic acids, phenol, low pH, and high phosphate and sodium chloride concentrations, all inhibiting motility of *Bdellovibrio* cells, were found concomitantly to inhibit attachment. The close association of attachment to motility is further supported by the lack of motility and attachment under anaerobic conditions and in the presence of azide (14).

Whether host substances exert chemotactic effects on *Bdellovibrio* merits further study. Some such mechanism is suggested by the observation that bdellovibrios seem to avoid nonsusceptible microorganisms in mixtures with host bacteria (17, 18). A direct demonstration of chemotactic attraction of bdellovibrios, as in J. Adler's classical studies on chemoreception in *Escherichia coli* (19), would provide critical information on whether the parasites can "sense" host substances. Such studies, as well as other details of the attachment phase, might well be facilitated by the use of conditional lethal, temperature-sensitive mutants recently isolated in our laboratory, which grow at 26 but not at 35 C. Some of these mutants are defective in their attachment capability at the higher temperature though they remain motile, perhaps because they have lost chemotactic responsiveness.

Normal changes in the physiological state of the host do not seem to influence attachment. In synchronized host cultures, bacteria at any stage of growth are susceptible to attachment of and penetration by bdellovibrios.

What are the host-cell properties requisite for parasite attachment, and thus for determining the host range of the parasite? This question can be studied at the molecular level, using host cell-wall mutants with defined deficiencies in cell-wall composition. Series of mutants of several species of Enterobacteriaceae with progressive blocks in the biosynthesis of cell-wall lipopolysaccharides (LPS) are indeed available. Using these mutants as hosts, it was possible to define the receptor sites for *Bdellovibrio* attachment, as determined by the rate and percent of attachment. Rough strains of *Salmonella* and *E. coli,* having a complete LPS core but lacking the repeating sugar units (type specific O antigens), yield better attachment rates than the respective smooth wild types with complete cores and outer repeating units, or than the more extreme rough mutants with deficiencies in the polysaccharide core. The complete LPS cell-wall core thus appears to constitute a suitable binding site for the parasite. The LPS core is common to the cell walls of Enterobacteriaceae and may thus explain their similar abilities to serve as receptors for bdellovibrios, i.e., the broad range of gram-negative hosts. The inhibition of attachment observed in smooth types may be a nonspecific masking effect by the outer sugar units (20).

A similar nonspecific protective effect of a cell-wall protein layer in *Spirillum serpens* has been described (21). *Bdellovibrio*-resistant strains of this bacterium possess a regularly arranged and closely packed single-protein layer on the cell-wall surface. When the protein was removed, the bacterium was rendered sensitive to *Bdellovibrio* attachment, and when the protein was allowed to reassemble on the host cell wall, *Bdellovibrio* no longer attached to the host bacterium.

The physiological condition of the host cell affects penetration. The physical approximation of the host's cytoplasmic membrane to the parasite's attachment pole has been suggested to be obligatory for penetration, so that plasmolyzed or aged bacteria, in which the membrane is withdrawn from the cell wall, are not penetrated (11).

Penetration is blocked by inhibitors of protein synthesis such as puromycin, streptomycin and chloramphenicol (22). Experiments with streptomycin-resistant *Bdellovibrio* and host mutants indicated that the inhibitor acts on the parasite. It is possible that certain inducible enzymes have to be formed by the parasite for dissolution of the host's wall and subsequent invasion. The presumed inducers might well be located within the host's cell wall where the binding sites are located, and might act upon the *Bdellovibrio* only when unmasked by direct contact.

Early damage to the host after attachment and penetration was demonstrated by measurement of respiration rate and the rate of the hydrolysis of orthonitrophenyl galactoside (ONPG) in cryptic mutants of *E. coli* (ML 35) which lack permease for β-galactosides, but have constitutive galactosidase (12). During a single infection cycle, there is early increased permeability of the host membrane. The initial sharp increase in O_2 uptake with lactose as substrate declines to extinction with equal rapidity. The rapid onset of these effects and the fact that streptomycin does not fully prevent damage to the host, indicate that the host's cytoplasmic membrane is damaged even before complete penetration by the parasite.

Protein, DNA and RNA synthesis in the host cease within minutes after exposure to the parasite (22). This is well demonstrated in the inhibition of inducible galactosidase synthesis in preinduced *E. coli,* which begins 3 to 5 min after infection. The enzyme production continues to slow down and cease altogether after another 18 to 20 min. The kinetics of the inhibition of enzyme synthesis by infection resemble those obtained when the inducer is removed from the preinducer system. It thus seems possible that this inhibition involves an effect on enzyme-specific RNA formation. When *E. coli* host cells are exposed to *Bdellovibrio* and inducer simultaneously, hardly any enzyme is synthesized.

By employing a system in which host and *Bdellovibrio* had widely different DNA base ratios and analyzing their respective DNA on CsCl gradients, it was recently found in Rittenberg's laboratory (personal communication) that the host's DNA is broken down before the parasite accomplishes significant DNA synthesis of its own.

Nature of the nutritional factors and conditions, provided by the host, upon which the parasite depends. Bdellovibrio does not require a living host for its growth and development. An obligate parasitic *Bdellovibrio* strain was found to grow and multiply within UV-killed or heat-treated (70 C) *E. coli* cells. This strain was also found to regenerate its flagellum and incorporate amino acids in the usual growth medium in the absence of host cells (Varon and Kessel, personal communication). Furthermore, *Bdellovibrio* does not depend on its host for energy-supplying mechanisms. Host-dependent (HD) parasite strains have the enzymatic capacities (aldolase, glyceraldehyde-3-phosphate dehydrogenase, pyruvate kinase and lactate dehydrogenase) for obtaining energy from substrate-linked phosphorylations. They also process a complete tricarboxylic acid cycle, contain succinate dehydrogenase in their particulate fraction, have a cytochrome system and even show enhanced respiration in the presence of a few exogenous substrates (23).

An important step in the elucidation of the nutritional basis of the parasitic interaction of *Bdellovibrio* with its host was the isolation of host-independent derivatives (HID) which retain their facultative parasitic capacities (24, 25). Such HID strains have also been isolated with relatively high frequency by Seidler and Starr (26) and should not be confused with the nonmotile, nonparasitic *Bdellovibrio* mutants (HI) isolated by Stolp and Starr (27). The facultative parasitic (HID) *Bdellovibrio* mutants form colonies on solid media in the absence of host cells and also produce plaques on host lawns. They grow especially well on complex media containing protein digests and yeast extracts and on host cells in suspension. Growth-initiating factors are required to start development in host-free media when small inocula are used (24).

Since the HID can be obtained from the wild-type parasites at relatively high frequency, only a few genetic loci appear to be involved in determining the absolute dependence on host, and only a few host factors may be absolutely required by wild-type *Bdellovibrio*.

A systematic study was therefore undertaken to isolate host factors which would allow for the development and multiplication of obligate HD *Bdellovibrio* strains in host-free systems and thus simulate the endoparasitic state. In specific conditions, a certain portion of wild-type (HD) bdellovibrios grew well and divided in media containing cell-free extracts (or "factors") of different microorganisms (28). Under these conditions, part of the *Bdellovibrio* population developed into extremely long, nonmotile coils which resembled those observed in host-free cultures of HID *Bdellovibrio* strains (13). Under conditions of elevated osmotic pressure, these (HD + factor) coils fragment into progeny units (up to 100 units per coil). It thus seems that a variety of environmental factors in the host's periplasm, including the attainment of critical concentrations of certain growth factors in this microenvironment, may be as important as the gross nutritional requirements for host dependency.

The factor in the cellular extracts of different microorganisms which induces formation of long coils is nondialyzable and is stable to deoxyribonuclease and pronase (28), but is highly sensitive to ribonuclease Aviva Horovitz, personal communication).

Until recently, the long coils of *Bdellovibrio* were thought to develop exclusively in host-free systems. However, recent studies in our laboratory, using different-sized host cells, showed that long coils can develop within giant host filaments. There is a direct correlation between the volume of the host cell and the size of the *Bdellovibrio* coil, the final number of parasite progeny, and the time required for completion of the life cycle. Using *E. coli* strains and their mutants which form coenocytic giant filaments, it was found that extremely long coils, which continue to grow as long as host protoplasm is available, develop in the giant filaments and finally produce from 50 to 100 progeny after 6 to 8 hr. Only four to seven progeny are produced in normal-sized hosts whose entire cycle is completed within 2 hr. In *E. coli* cells of intermediate sizes, intermediate progeny numbers and cycle intervals are observed. This relationship of parasite development and division to cell volume may shed light on the conditions which trigger division in *Bdellovibrio*.

The morphological similarities of bdellovibrios developing as parasites

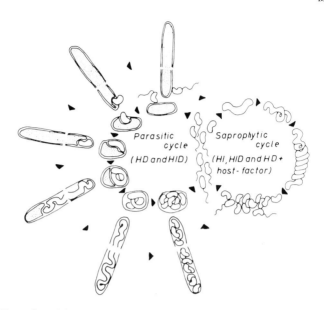

FIG. 1.   Life cycles of bdellovibrios within and without host cells.
The parasitic cycles, shown on the left, involve development of the same *Bdello-vibrio* strain within normal-sized *E. coli* hosts (inner circle) and within giant coenocytic *E. coli* filaments (outer circle). Such parasitic life cycles are observed with HD and certain HID strains (24, 26).
The saprophytic life cycle of bdellovibrios, shown on the right, can be observed in HID strains, in HI strains (26), as well as in host-free cultures of HD strains grown in the presence of a "host factor" (HD + factor) (28).

within host cells and growing independently of the host (HID as well as HD + factor) are indicated schematically in Fig. 1 (based on the scheme of Burnham et al., 13).

Evolution of the parasitic state. The taxonomic creation of the *Bdellovibrio* genus by Stolp and Starr (29) was based solely on the predatory character of the bacteria. However, later observations have raised doubts as to whether this group is indeed homogeneous.

Studies of DNA base compositions of a number of *Bdellovibrio* strains showed that there are at least two distinct *Bdellovibrio* groupings: those with 43% GC and those with 50 to 52.3% GC (30). Other differential characters related to these two groups are sensitivity to antibiotics and the formation of exocellular protease.

Bdellovibrio-like organisms, isolated by Guelin and Sisman (31), cause lysis of *Clostridium perfringens* and *C. histolyticum,* and seem to penetrate the host. Some of these organisms are pleomorphic, do not seem to possess flagella and are not obligate parasites.

These findings imply that *Bdellovibrio* parasitism is not a single isolated case, but is a more general phenomenon and may involve several parallel lines of microbial evolution.

The *Bdellovibrio* parasitic system is highly complex, displaying specialized organelles, complicated attachment and penetration mechanisms and specific nutritional requirements. In order to cast light on its evolution, it would be of interest to find examples of bacterial groups capable of attacking and lysing other microorganisms which have more primitive and less complex modes of interaction with their hosts. One such example might be found in a myxobacter isolated in our laboratory (32), which specifically lyses vegetative cells of blue-green algae, but not algal heterocytes. None of these myxobacteria is an obligate parasite, and penetration of the host does not seem to occur. As with *Bdellovibrio*, however, lysis of the hosts is accomplished only upon direct polar contact of the myxobacteria with the host, after an interval of several minutes of contact. The myxobacteria lack specific attachment organelles, and are capable of lysing hosts only on solid medium. Lysis does not take place in liquid media, including shaken cultures, even containing extremely high numbers of organisms.

REFERENCES

1. FULTON JD. Metabolism and pathogenic mechanisms of parasitic protozoa. *Res Protozool* **3**: 398–504, 1969.
2. MOULDER JW. A model for studying the biology of parasitism: *Chlamydia psittaci* in L cells. *Bio Science* **19**: 875–881, 1969.
3. BUCHNER P. "Endosymbiosis of animals with plant microorganisms." New York, Interscience Publishers, John Wiley & Sons, Inc, 1965.
4. HALL WT and CLAUS G. Ultrastructural studies on the blue-green algal symbiont in *Cyanophora paradoxa* Kroschikoff. *J Cell Biol* **19**: 551–563, 1963.
5. CHAPMAN-ANDERSEN C and HOLTER H. Respiration in *Pelomyxa palustris*. *J Protozool* **16**: 30, 1969.
6. STANIER RY. Some aspects of the biology of cells and their possible evolutionary significance. *Symp Soc Gen Microbiol* **20**: 1–38, 1970.
7. STOLP H and PETZHOLD H. Untersuchungen über einen obligat parasitischen Mikroorganismus mit lytischer Activität für Pseudomonas Bakterien. *Phytopathology* **45**: 364–390, 1962.
8. SHILO M. Morphological and physiological aspects of the interaction of *Bdellovibrio* with host bacteria. *Curr Top Microbiol Immunol* **50**: 174–204, 1969.
9. ABRAM D and DAVIS BK. Structural properties and features of parasitic *Bdellovibrio bacteriovorus*. *J Bacteriol* **104**: 948–965, 1970.
10. BURNHAM JC, HASHIMOTO T and CONTI SF. Electron microscopic observa-

12 M. SHILO

tions on the penetration of *Bdellovibrio bacteriovorus* into gram-negative bacterial hosts. *J Bacteriol* **96**: 1366–1381, 1968.

11. ABRAM D and CHOU D. Mechanism of entry into host cells by *Bdellovibrio bacteriovorus*. *Bacteriol Proc* **G**: 121, 1971.

12. RITTENBERG SC and SHILO M. Early host damage in the infection cycle of *Bdellovibrio bacteriovorus*. *J Bacteriol* **102**: 149–169, 1970.

13. BURNHAM JC, HASHIMOTO T and CONTI SF. Ultrastructure and cell division of a facultatively parasitic strain of *Bdellovibrio bacteriovorus*. *J Bacteriol* **101**: 997–1004, 1970.

14. VARON M and SHILO M. Interaction of *Bdellovibrio bacteriovorus* and host bacteria. I. Kinetic studies of attachment and invasion of *E. coli* B by *Bdellovibrio bacteriovorus* 109, *J Bacteriol* **95**: 744–753, 1968.

15. VARON M and SHILO M. Interaction of *Bdellovibrio bacteriovorus* and host bacteria. II. Intracellular growth and development of *Bdellovibrio bacteriovorus* strain 109 in liquid cultures. *J Bacteriol* **99**: 136–141, 1969.

16. SEIDLER RJ and STARR MP. Factors affecting the intracellular parasitic growth of *Bdellovibrio bacteriovorus* developing within *Escherichia coli*. *J Bacteriol* **97**: 912–923, 169.

17. STARR MP and BAIGNANT NL. Parasitic interaction of *Bdellovibrio bacteriovorus* with other bacteria. *J Bacteriol* **91**: 2006–2017, 1966.

18. STOLP M. "Lysis von Bakterien durch den Parasiten *Bdellovibrio bacteriovorus*." Göttingen, Institut für den wissenschaftlichen Film, 1967.

19. ADLER J. Chemoreception in bacteria. *Science* **166**: 1588–1597, 1969.

20. VARON M and SHILO M. Attachment of *Bdellovibrio bacteriovorus* to cell wall mutants of *Salmonella* and *Escherichia coli*. *J Bacteriol* **97**: 977–979, 1969.

21. BUCKMIRE FLA. A protective role for a cell wall protein layer of *Spirillum serpens* against infection by *Bdellovibrio bacteriovorus*. *Bacteriol Proc* **G**: 122, 1971.

22. VARON M, DRUCKER I and SHILO M. Early effects of *Bdellovibrio bacteriovorus* infection on the syntheses of protein and RNA of host bacteria. *Biochem Biophys Res Commun* **37**: 518, 1969.

23. SIMPSON FJ and ROBINSON J. Some energy-producing systems in *Bdellovibrio bacteriovorus* strains 6–5S. *Can J Biochem* **46**: 865–873, 1968.

24. SHILO M and BRUFF B. Lysis of gram negative bacteria by host-independent ectoparasitic *Bdellovibrio bacteriovorus* isolates. *J Gen Microbiol* **40**: 317–328, 1965.

25. DIETRICH DL, DENNY CF, HASHIMOTO T and CONTI SF. Facultatively parasitic strain of *Bdellovibrio bacteriovorus*. *J Bacteriol* **101**: 989–996, 1970.

26. SEIDLER RJ and STARR MP. Isolation and characterization of host-independent bdellovibrios. *J Bacteriol* **100**: 769–785, 1969.

27. STOLP H and STARR MP. Bacteriolysis. *Annu Rev Microbiol* **19**: 79–102, 1965.

28. REINER AM and SHILO M. Host-independent growth of *Bdellovibrio bacteriovorus* in microbial extracts. *J Gen Microbiol* **59**: 401–410, 1969.

29. STOLP H and STARR MP. Bdellovibrio bacteriovorus gen et sp n, a predatory ectoparasitic and bacteriolytic microorganism. *Antonie van Leeuwenhoek* **29**: 217–248, 1963.

30. SEIDLER RJ, STARR MP and MANDEL M. Deoxyribonucleic acid characterization of bdellovibrios. *J Bacteriol* **100**: 786–790, 1969.

31. GUELIN A and SISMAN J. Isolement de l'eau de rivière d'un parasite du bacille typhique. *Izv Akad Nauk SSSR [Biol]* **3**: 395–401, 1968.

32. SHILO M. Lysis of blue-green algae by myxobacter. *J Bacteriol* **104**: 453–461, 1970.

MOLECULAR ASPECTS OF THE INTERACTION OF MAMMALIAN CELLS WITH OBLIGATE MICROBIAL PARASITES AND VIRAL AGENTS

YECHIEL BECKER

Laboratory for Molecular Virology, Department of Virology,
Hebrew University–Hadassah Medical School, Jerusalem, Israel

INTRODUCTION

Mammalian cells *in vivo* and *in vitro* can be parasitized by obligate parasites of microbial and viral nature. Such infection may have different consequences for the infected host cells: a) the cells may act against the invading agents and prevent their ability to replicate; b) cell macromolecular processes may be inhibited, leading to cell death; and c) the cells and the parasites may reach an equilibrium, at least for a certain period after infection, during which both cells and parasite can continue to synthesize macromolecules. This latter circumstance may lead to changes in the control of macromolecular processes which can, in turn, give rise to uncontrolled growth by the infected cells. The schematic analysis of the results of host cell-parasite interaction indicates that both the host and the parasite are intimately involved in the processes which result from infection, and that the condition of the cell as well of the parasite can control the outcome of such interaction.

It is not surprising that mammalian cells respond profoundly to infection with obligate parasites, in view of the common presence in nature of biological entities which depend on the cell for the propagation of their genetic material. Such entities, by definition obligate parasites, require the host cell for the provision of nutrients which they cannot synthesize, or for biochemical processes which they lack. Their requirements as obligate parasites differ markedly. The chlamydiae are prokaryotic infectious particles, which contain both the DNA genome and ribosomal

This paper was written while the author was a National Science Foundation Senior Scientist at the Department of Microbiology, University of Chicago, Chicago, Ill.

[13]

subunits and enzymes, whereas viruses carry only the DNA or RNA genome, which depends on host cell ribosomes for the translation of its genetic messages. Since the biochemical requirements of different parasites differ from one another, it is to be expected that the reaction of the host cell to infection with various prokaryotic and viral agents also differs markedly. In the present study, we shall focus our attention on two models of host-parasite interactions and on the consequences of such infections. The trachoma agent and herpes simplex (HS) and Epstein-Barr (EB) viruses were chosen because of the variety of molecular processes which take place as a result of the interaction of these agents with the mammalian host cell.

Trachoma agent is an obligate prokaryotic parasite of the human eye which currently causes a chronic disease in about 400 million people throughout the world. HS virus is also widespread and is known to cause diseases in human beings apparently involving nerves of both the central and peripheral nervous systems. At the same time, it is a typical latent virus, which can be activated in the human body by hormonal changes. In addition, a herpes virus, the EB virus, appears to be causally involved in human cancer and may be able to transform human leukocytes. In order to study the molecular processes which accompany the interaction of individual host cells with an obligate parasite, our investigations were performed on cells cultured *in vitro*. Although it is not easy to correlate phenomena thus observed to the response of the infected cells *in vivo*, it is permissible to assume that the molecular processes at the cellular level are at least similar *in vitro* and *in vivo*. The description of the molecular processes of host-parasite interaction presented here is based largely on these studies, which provide a broad picture of different aspects of host-parasite interaction.

MOLECULAR COMPOSITION OF THE OBLIGATE PARASITES, TRACHOMA AGENT AND HERPES VIRUS AND OF HOST CELLS

The two parasites which were studied belong to two groups of biological agents: a) The trachoma agent is a member of the chlamydiae group of microorganisms. The infectious particle (designated elementary body) is a cellular entity (prokaryocyte) which lacks the ability to develop outside of the mammalian host cell. Upon infection of a mammalian cell, the trachoma elementary bodies develop into larger structures, which also retain their cellular characteristics. b) The herpes virions exist outside the host cell as particles consisting of protein and lipoprotein coats, apparently protecting the DNA genome. The genetic material of the virus can replicate only inside a mammalian cell. Upon infection of a host cell, the viral DNA genomes exist as naked nucleic acid molecules, and the virus growth cycle is terminated when the viral genomes are again coated.

Both trachoma and herpes virus affect the host cell as a result of their replicative processes. In order to understand the mechanisms of these processes, it is necessary to explore the organization and the nature of the genetic information present in the two parasites.

Molecular structure of trachoma agent infectious elementary bodies. The infectious unit of trachoma agent is an oval particle with a diameter of 0.3 μ. Electron microscopic analysis of the particles shows a rigid cell wall, an electron-dense nucleoid and ribosomal subunits in the cytoplasm of the particles (1).

In order to analyze the nature of the macromolecules which compose the trachoma elementary bodies, a synthetic medium was developed which supports the development of trachoma agent in infected cells (2). Different radioisotopes can be added to the culture medium of the infected cells. These are utilized for the synthesis of the trachoma macromolecules during the growth cycle and are incorporated into the trachoma elementary bodies. The latter are purified by centrifugation in sucrose gradients and then subjected to various molecular analyses.

1) DNA: Treatment of trachoma elementary bodies with detergents and the proteolytic enzyme pronase released the DNA molecules which were then analyzed (3). The genome of trachoma agent was found to be a circular DNA molecule, with a contour length of 330 μ and a molecular weight of 660×10^6 daltons. Such a DNA molecule is about 1/4 the size of *E. coli* DNA genome, and may contain genes for the synthesis of several hundred different proteins.

2) RNA: Analysis of the RNA present in the trachoma elementary bodies by zone centrifugation in sucrose gradients (4) or by electrophoresis on acrylamide gels (4a) demonstrated the occurrence of ribosomal and nonribosomal RNA species. The 50 S and 30 S ribosomal subunits present in the elementary bodies contain 23 S and 16 S RNA, respectively. In addition, 4 S RNA molecules, probably tRNA, and 5 S RNA molecules were obtained (Fig. 1).

3) Ribosomal subunits: Zone centrifugation in sucrose gradients of the cytoplasmic extracts, obtained from the deoxycholate-treated trachoma

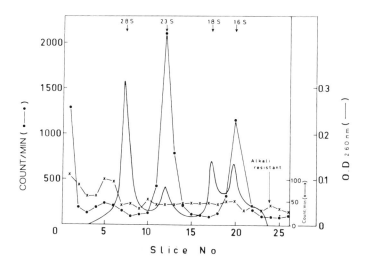

FIG. 1. Characterization of trachoma agent RNA by electrophoresis in acrylamide gels.

FL cells (derived from human amnion) were infected with trachoma agent and by centrifugation in sucrose gradients and the RNA was extracted by treatment labeled with H3-cytidine for 48 hr. The trachoma elementary bodies were purified with sodium dodecyl sulfate (SDS) buffer (Tris 0.005 M, NaCl 0.1 M, pH 7.3, SDS 0.5%) and analyzed by electrophoresis for 4 hr (5 mamp per gel) in 3% acrylamide gels. The OD_{260nm} profile (———) shows ribosomal RNA obtained from mammalian (FL) cells having sedimentation constants of 28 and 18 Svedberg units as well as ribosomal RNA from *E. coli* with S values of 23 and 16.

The trachoma agent RNA (•———•) (radioactivity determined as count/min) appeared in those regions of the gel where RNA with sedimentation constants of 23 and 16 Svedberg units would concentrate. To demonstrate that the 23 and 16 S molecules were RNA and not DNA, one gel was treated with KOH for 18 hr at 37 C after which the remaining trichloroacetic acid-precipitable radioactivity (alkali-resistant radioactivity X———X was determined.

elementary bodies, showed the presence of ribosomal subunits with sedimentation coefficients of 50 S and 30 S, respectively (4). The larger subunits contain 23 S RNA molecules while the 30 S particles contain 16 S RNA molecules. The presence of such subunits, but absence of complete ribosomes, in the trachoma elementary bodies even in high Mg^{2+} concentrations indicates that the infectious particle lacks the conditions which enable the formation of active ribosomes. It is possible that the formation of ribosomes cannot take place in the absence of mRNA molecules. The stimulation of mRNA synthesis in the elementary bodies

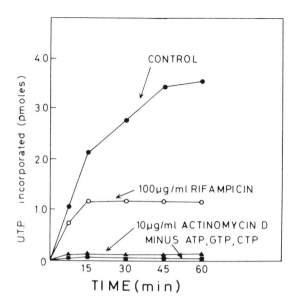

FIG. 2. RNA synthesis *in vitro* by trachoma DNA-dependent RNA polymerase. The complete system contained the following components (in μmoles) in a final volume of 0.2 ml: Mg^{++}, 0.8; Mn^{++}, 0.2; 2-mercaptoethanol, 0.2; Tris-HCl, pH 7.5, 10; adenosine triphosphate (ATP), cytosine triphosphate (CTP) and guanosine triphosphate (GTP) each 0.008; H^3-uridine triphosphate (UTP) 0.003. To 0.1 ml of this solution was added 0.1 ml containing the following: 2 to 5×10^7 purified trachoma elementary bodies ($\sim$ 2 to 5 μg of protein) prepared in 0.1 M Tris-HCl, pH 7.5, containing 8% (w/w) sucrose; 10^{-3} M 2-mercaptoethanol and 10^{-3} M Mg^{++}.

The complete reaction mixture was incubated at 36 C and samples were removed every 15 min. The reaction was stopped by the addition of 1 ml of ice-cold 10% (w/w) trichloroacetic acid (TCA) containing 0.3% (w/w) NaH_2PO_4. The suspension was kept at 4 C for 10 min and then filtered through Millipore filters and washed with 30 ml of 10% TCA containing 0.3% NaH_2PO_4. The filters were dried and the radioactivity was counted in a Packard liquid scintillation counter. The complete reaction mixture incorporated H^3-UTP into RNA chains. However, after treatment with actinomycin D (10 μg/ml) (which binds to the DNA template), the reaction was completely inhibited. Similarly, no reaction took place in the absence of ATP, GTP and CTP. When the reaction mixture was treated with rifampicin (100 μg/ml), RNA synthesis continued during the initial 15 min and was then completely inhibited.

after their entry into the cytoplasm of a mammalian cell might enable the ribosomal subunits to associate with the mRNA and to initiate its translation.

4) DNA-dependent RNA polymerase: The elementary bodies of the trachoma agent represent its dormant phase and are capable of surviving outside the host cell. A specific DNA-dependent RNA polymerase is present in the elementary bodies which can be activated by the addition of ATP, GTP, CTP and UTP (5). About 60% of the enzyme molecules are bound to the DNA molecule, most probably in an initiated form, as indicated by their resistance to rifampicin treatment (Fig. 2). Under conditions which permit the transcription of the trachoma DNA, the enzyme molecules synthesize RNA molecules of high molecular weight (6). The high sensitivity of trachoma agent to rifampicin (7) is due to the ability of the antibiotic to irreversibly inhibit the RNA polymerase (8).

5) Protein compositon of the elementary bodies: Analysis of the proteins labeled with radioactive amino acids present in the elementary bodies by electrophoresis on acrylamide gels demonstrated 40 different proteins (9). Staining of the gels disclosed only 19 protein bands (Fig. 3). Most of these proteins probably compose the ribosomal subunits of the trachoma agent and each band may contain several different proteins of similar molecular weight.

We can conclude from these incomplete data that the elementary body of the trachoma agent has the features of a prokaryotic cell (10), a property which clearly distinguishes it from the viruses.

Molecular composition of herpes virions. The main feature which characterizes the herpes virion, as well as all other viruses, is the lack of cellular organization. Essentially, the virion is composed of a genome made of a nucleic acid molecule (double stranded DNA in the case of HS virus), which contains all the genetic information needed for the replication of the virus. In certain viruses (pox virions), an enzyme is present in the virion which is capable of transcribing the early viral mRNA (11). In others (leukemia viruses), an enzyme has been described which transcribes DNA from a single stranded RNA (12, 13). The nature of this enzyme and its molecular product are still unknown. Other viruses may depend on host cell processes for the initial expression of their genetic information. DNA-dependent RNA polymerase activity was not found in the herpes virions.

1) DNA: The genome of HS virus is packed inside a capsid which has a diameter of 80 nm and is composed of 162 hollow, cylindrical capsomeres arranged in icosahedral symmetry (14). The capsid is covered with three lipid envelopes which increase the diameter of the virion to 110 nm (15). Treatment of the enveloped virions with detergents and

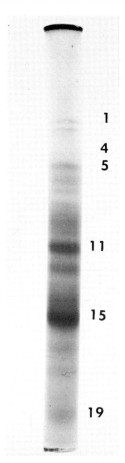

FIG. 3. Characterization of trachoma agent proteins by electrophoresis in acrylamide gels.

Trachoma elementary bodies purified by centrifugation in sucrose gradients were dissolved with sodium dodecyl sulfate, urea and 2-mercaptoethanol and boiled for 2 min. They were then subjected to electrophoresis for 20 hr (6 mamp per gel) in 10% (w/w) acrylamide gels. The gels were stained with 0.5% (w/v) amido black, decolorized with 7.5% (v/v) acetic acid and photographed. Approximately 20 separate protein bands can be resolved by this method.

pronase makes possible the isolation of intact HS viral DNA genomes. The length of the DNA molecules is about 50 μ and the molecular weight of the DNA about 100×10^6 daltons. A similar value was obtained by zone centrifugation in sucrose gradients together with vaccinia DNA molecules employed as a marker (16). The HS viral DNA has a G + C

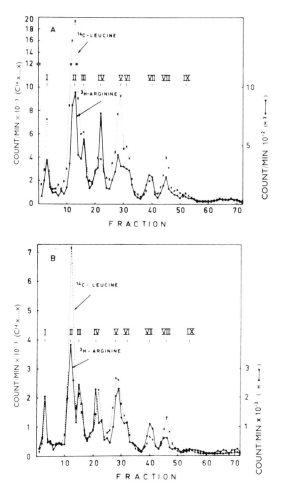

FIG. 4. Acrylamide gel electrophorograms of enveloped herpes virions. Enveloped virus particles, labeled with radioactive leucine and arginine, were obtained from the nuclear (Fig. 4A) and cytoplasmic (Fig. 4B) fractions of BSC_1 (green monkey kidney) cells infected with HS virus and incubated at 37 C for 18 hr. The enveloped virions were obtained from each fraction by zone centrifugation in sucrose gradients (12 to 52% w/w) for 40 min at 24,000 rev/min using the SW 25.1 rotor of the L–2 Beckman preparative ultracentrifuge at 7 C. The virus bands containing enveloped virions were removed and centrifuged at $100,000 \times g$ for 1 hr. The virus pellet was dissolved in sodium dodecyl sulfate, urea and 2-mercaptoethanol, and analyzed by acrylamide gel electrophoresis.

Nine proteins were demonstrated in the coat of mature HS virions. The molecular weight of these proteins ranged from 140,000 (protein I) to 24,000 (protein IX) daltons. The major constituent of the herpes virion is protein II (mol wt 110,000 content of about 60% and a density of 1.720 g/ml, and contains genetic information for the synthesis of a large number of different proteins (assuming that all the DNA contains genetic information).

2) Structural coat proteins: Analysis of purified HS virions by acryl-amide gel electrophoresis disclosed the presence of 12 major proteins in the viral capsid and envelopes (17). The isolation of empty capsids and of partially enveloped and fully enveloped virions from infected cells, which were labeled with radioactive amino acids, made it possible to determine the site and role of each protein in the viral coat (Fig. 4). Two proteins (II and VIII) compose the capsid, two (VI, VII) are the internal proteins, rich in arginine, and proteins III, IV and V are glycoproteins present in the three viral envelopes. The envelope glycoproteins are coded by HS virus and made during the virus growth cycle, whereas the lipid moiety of the viral envelopes is of cellular origin and is made in the cell prior to infection (18). The nature of proteins I and IX to XII is still under analysis.

These findings indicate that the herpes virion is organized in a complex and specific way, but still lacks cellular organization. Indeed, the viral DNA genomes can function only when present in the infected cell as uncoated molecules. It thus appears that the viral DNA depends on the host cell for the expression of its genetic information, both for transcription (synthesis of early viral mRNA) and translation (of viral mRNA species by the cellular ribosomes).

Molecular aspects of the mammalian cell. The mammalian cell is a highly complicated structure which contains at least a million genes organized in the different chromosomal DNA molecules. The latter are organized within the nucleus, a distinct compartment in the cell, separated by a membrane from the cytoplasm, which is also limited by the cellular membrane.

The life cycle of the cell is divided into several phases, during which various molecular processes take place. The S phase is characterized as that during which the chromosomal DNA and part of the mitochondrial DNA are duplicated. The G2 phase is the period of active RNA and protein synthesis which is terminated by cell division (mitosis), and the G1 phase occurs prior to, and represents a preparation for, the S phase.

daltons). Certain proteins were found to be richer in arginine than others. The arginine-rich proteins include proteins I, III, IV, VI and VII, the latter having the highest ratio of arginine to leucine.

It is clearly impossible to describe in detail all the processes which take place in the eukaryotic cell, and only those molecular events which are essential for an understanding of the host-parasite interaction will be briefly described.

1) RNA synthesis: Most of the cellular RNA synthesis takes place in the nuclei. The ribosomal precursor RNA (19) is transcribed by a specific RNA polymerase (20) in the nucleoli. The RNA is methylated and processed into distinct molecules, which are coated by ribosomal proteins and form the ribosomal subunits. The latter are transported from the nuclei to the cytoplasm. In addition, tRNA, as well as mRNA molecules, are transcribed from the chromosomal DNA. Both RNA species are transported from the nuclei to the cytoplasm, where they function in protein synthesis.

2) Protein synthesis: Studies on the fate of the nascent mRNA and ribosomal subunits indicate that the ribosomal subunits interact with the mRNA molecules (21) to form active ribosomes on which proteins are synthesized (22). The mechanism of mRNA translation by ribosomes has been described in detail (23).

The cultured cell lines used for the studies on host-parasite interaction are nonsynchronized. The molecular analyses thus represent values which are average values for the culture cells in different stages of their life cycle. Therefore, in order to distinguish the molecular processes of the parasite from those of the cells, conditions were selected which permit differentiation between the cellular and the viral macromolecules.

INTERACTION OF OBLIGATE PARASITES WITH THE HOST CELL

The initial phase of the interaction of obligate parasites with the host cell is their attachment to the cell membrane, an electrostatic process which results from the collision of the particles with the cell membrane. The particles which interact with the cell may either be repelled or become attached to the cell membrane, and engulfment of the attached parasite into the host cell cytoplasm may follow. The kinetics of these processes has been studied with both the trachoma agent and herpes virions (24, 25).

  Trachoma agent: interaction and entry into the host cell. Addition of purified labeled trachoma elementary bodies to cultured BSC₁ cells (a line of kidney cells derived from an African green monkey kidney cell culture) results in the gradual attachment of elementary bodies to the cell membrane. Within 3 hr, all the particles which are capable of interacting with the cells are attached to their surfaces (24). The particles enter the cytoplasm during the absorption period, and most probably also during the next few hours. Electron microscopic studies on the process of cell infection with trachoma elementary bodies (24) suggest that the particle is introduced into the host cell cytoplasm by a process of pinocytosis. Within the host cell cytoplasm, the elementary bodies reach the Golgi region in the vicinity of the nuclear membrane. It is not yet known if this cytoplasmic site is selected by the trachoma elementary bodies due to the availability in this region of essential metabolites, or whether the constant streaming of the cytoplasm is mechanically responsible for this localization of the particles.

The trachoma elementary bodies which enter the host cell cytoplasm retain their cellular structure throughout the developmental cycle. The initial process which has been detected in the elementary body is the synthesis of RNA (26), most probably by the DNA-dependent RNA polymerase present in the elementary bodies (5). Development of the elementary bodies into inclusion bodies is initiated only 6 hr after infection.

HS virus: interaction and entry into the cell. The kinetics of interaction of purified HS virions with the cell membrane were studied with the aid of purified virions. That the virions interact with the host cell membrane in an electrostatic manner was suggested by the observation that heparin, a negatively charged molecule, caused the detachment of virions which had previously been attached to the surface of the cell membrane, but did not affect virus particles already incorporated into the host cell cytoplasm. After entry into the cytoplasm, the herpes virions become associated with membranes (25). Electron microscopic studies suggest that the outer membrane of the virions may interact with the cell membrane during the absorption stage (15).

Within the host cell cytoplasm the herpes virions are uncoated by cellular enzymes. The coat proteins are retained in the cytoplasm, whereas the DNA molecules are gradually transported into the nuclei. The response of the cell to the penetration of the foreign particle thus releases the viral DNA and enables it to function. In this way the cell itself actively participates in a process which changes its fate (25).

Response of the host cell to infection. 1) Cellular effects on the parasites: The cell may interfere with infection by an obligate parasite by either rejecting the particles which attach to the cell membrane or by enzymatic action against particles already incorporated into the cytoplasm. Certain viruses, which lack an envelope (e.g., picorna viruses), attach to the cell membrane only at specific receptors. In the absence of such receptor sites, these virions cannot interact with the cell membrane and the cells cannot be infected. After the engulfment of foreign particles into the cytoplasm, the cell responds by mobilizing lysosomes, which contain enzymes capable of degrading the invader. These enzymes can modify the structure of both the trachoma agent and of the herpes virus particles, but these parasites are only partially degraded. The trachoma elementary bodies retain the capacity to incorporate nutrients from the cell, and the viral nucleic acid is released and attains a molecular conformation which permits its replication. In both cases, the cell responding to infection does not eliminate the parasites but rather conditions their development.

2) The synthesis of interferon: Another type of cellular response to an invader, which may be either an obligate parasite or a naked, double-stranded polynucleotide molecule (e.g., poly I:C) (27), is the synthesis by the cell of protein molecules termed interferons. Interferons act to inhibit the development of obligate parasites such as chlamydiae (28) or viruses (29). The cellular mechanism which triggers the synthesis of interferon molecules and their mode of action are not yet fully understood. However, interferon has been shown to trigger the synthesis of new protein molecules (29) which participate in the inhibition of the translation of viral mRNA. Viruses of various groups differ in their sensitivity to inhibition by interferon. Thus, whereas cytoplasmic viruses are generally highly sensitive, the nuclear DNA viruses (to which herpes viruses belong) are less sensitive.

MOLECULAR ASPECTS OF TRACHOMA INFECTION:
THE DEVELOPMENT OF A CHRONIC DISEASE

Under experimental conditions, cells infected with trachoma agent lack a mechanism controlling the development of this parasite. The enzymatic attack to which the elementary bodies are subjected in the host cytoplasm initiates their development and the fate of the cell is then determined by the nature of the developmental cycle of the parasite, its nutritional demands and the synthesis of parasite products which may interfere with normal cellular physiology. In order to understand the cell-trachoma relationship, the life cycle of the parasite as well as the molecular processes which take place in this cycle must be analyzed.

Developmental cycle of trachoma agent. 1) Morphology of the cytoplasmic mass into smaller bodies (secondary bodies). These contain the ribosomes. The secondary bodies (Fig. 5B) divide by a process of binary fission to yield two daughter structures, each somewhat larger than the final elementary bodies. The cytoplasm of these daughter particles is contracted, the DNA genome is condensed and the membrane of the particles becomes rigid due to the synthesis of a cell wall. At this stage, the structures are designated as the classic infectious elementary bodies. Molecular events in the trachoma cycle appear to support the morphological studies.

2) Morphology of the infected host cell: Observations of the ultrastructure of a cell infected with trachoma agent reveal that the cell nucleus is displaced from the center of the cell owing to the development of the large inclusion body. However, the nucleoli within the nucleus remain intact and most of the cytoplasmic organelles are retained, although they are displaced by the growing trachoma inclusion body. The developmental cycle of trachoma agent takes place within a period of 48 hr (the progeny of elementary bodies develop during the period of 24 to 48 hr after infection); and the host cell is probably affected only at the time when the inclusion bodies are filled with elementary bodies. Due to the mechanical effects of the large trachoma inclusion body, the infected cells rupture and the trachoma infectious elementary bodies are released.

Molecular processes during the developmental cycle of trachoma agent. 1) Initiation of RNA synthesis: With the aid of radioautography, it was demonstrated that the synthesis of RNA in the developing trachoma inclusion bodies is not dependent on RNA synthesis in the host cell nucleoli, and takes place in the developing trachoma structures (26). Furthermore, the trachoma RNA is synthesized by a specific RNA polymerase (5) which functions throughout most of the developmental cycle (30). RNA polymerase molecules in the elementary bodies can be initiated to synthesize RNA *in vitro* by incubation with the four nucleoside triphosphates, suggesting that the reason for the obligate parasitism of the trachoma agent is the need for a supply of the nucleoside triphosphates. The synthesis of RNA in the developing elementary bodies may make possible the initiation of the translational processes and the synthesis of proteins.

2) Trachoma protein synthesis: Analysis of the incorporation of radioactive amino acids by the trachoma-infected cells demonstrated that infection does not affect the synthesis of proteins (9). Similar results were

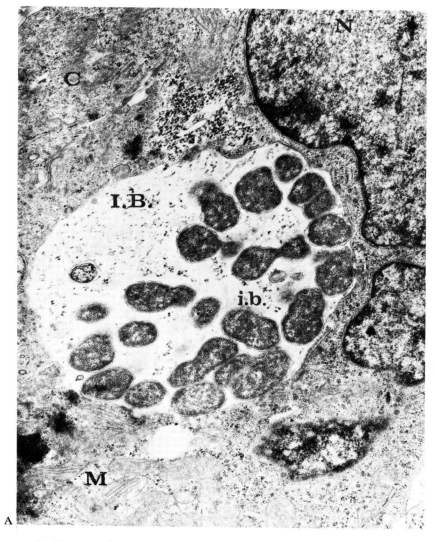

FIG. 5. Electron microscopy of the trachoma inclusion body.
FL cells, obtained from human amnion cells infected with the T'ang strain of trachoma agent, were fixed, sectioned, stained and examined in the JEM 7A electron microscope. Within the inclusion body, elementary bodies (0.3 μ) are synthesized from

obtained with cells infected with the meningopneumonitis agent (31). In order to distinguish between cellular and trachoma-protein synthesis, trachoma growth cycle: Study of the developmental cycle of the trachoma agent is based on electron microscopic examination of thin sections pre-

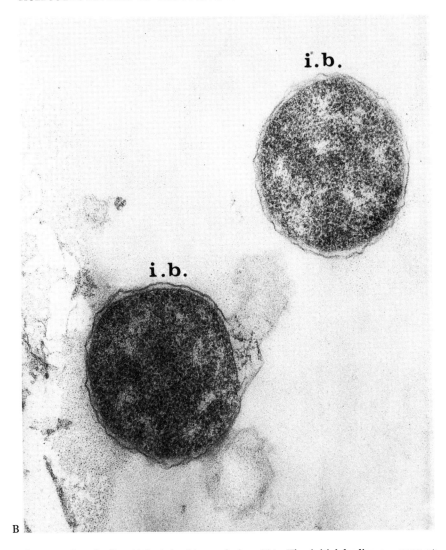

the secondary bodies (1.0 μ) by binary fission (A). The initial bodies are seen at
a higher magnification in (B). The small particles inside the bodies are the ribosomes.
× 17,500. N = Nucleus; C = Cytoplasm; M = Mitochondria; IB = Inclusion
body; ib = Initial (secondary) body.

pared from infected cells in the course of infection (Fig. 5). The trachoma
elementary body retains its cellular identity in the cytoplasm of the host
cell and develops into a large body (inclusion body) (Fig. 5A). Within
the inclusion bodies, membranes are synthesized which divide the parasite's

the infected cells were treated with cycloheximide, a potent inhibitor of protein synthesis in eukaryocytes, which does not affect prokaryotic cells. Under these conditions, about 90% of host protein synthesis was inhibited, while protein synthesis continued in the developing trachoma inclusions throughout the entire growth cycle of the agent (9, 31). The highest rate of protein synthesis occurs between 24 and 30 hr after infection, at the time when the initial infectious elementary bodies are being formed in the inclusion structures. The synthesis of these proteins was inhibited by rifampicin, a specific inhibitor of the trachoma agent. Different protein species were synthesized at different stages of the growth cycle (9).

Trimethoprim is an inhibitor of the enzyme which formylates methionyl tRNA. Since the trachoma agent is a prokaryotic cell in which the synthesis of peptide chains is initiated by formyl-methionyl-tRNA$_F$ (23), the effect of trimethoprim on the development of trachoma agent was studied. At concentrations of 10 to 100 μg/ml, for 24 hr prior to trachoma infection trimethoprim prevented the development of the agent in the treated cell.

3) Synthesis of trachoma nucleic acids: Trachoma RNA species, mostly 23 S and 16 S ribosomal RNA and tRNA, are synthesized in the developing inclusion bodies throughout the growth cycle of the agent. This RNA synthesis is inhibited by rifampicin.

Labeling of the infected cells with radioactive cytidine resulted in its incorporation into replicating DNA molecules. DNA molecules are synthesized at a low rate in the inclusion bodies during the first 30 hr of the growth cycle, However, an increased rate of DNA synthesis was observed at 36 hr, at the time when the number of elementary bodies rapidly increases. This sequence of macromolecular synthesis is in agreement with the morphological studies on the trachoma growth cycle.

Effect of trachoma infection on the host cell. The invading elementary bodies develop slowly in the cytoplasm of the host cell, without markedly affecting host cell processes. With the aid of rifampicin two populations of trachoma elementary bodies were distinguished: a) particles which initiate development after entry into the host cell and are inhibited by rifampicin; and b) particles which do not initiate RNA synthesis and are not affected by rifampicin. Not all the trachoma elementary bodies which penetrate into the cell can apparently initiate development. Some may remain latent in the cytoplasm of the infected cell, and develop only at a later stage. The possibility that the cell may interfere actively with the development of trachoma elementary bodies cannot be ruled out. As prokaryotic cells, the developing trachoma agents utilize their own ribosomes and enzymatic processes for the synthesis of macromolecules and depend on the host cells only for some of their metabolites. The extent of the parasitism is not yet known. It seems, however, that the host cell is affected only during the late stages of the developmental cycle. Details of the effects which lead to the eventual disintegration of the host cell and the release of the infectious elementary bodies are not yet known.

Similar processes appear to occur in the conjunctival cells of human eyes infected with trachoma agent. The agent develops slowly and at a localized site, and the elementary bodies infect neighboring cells, thus leading to a prolonged and chronic infection of the eye. As a result of damage to the conjunctival cells blood vessels penetrate into the infected tissue and a panus develops at the site of infection. The conjunctival tissue frequently cannot overcome the infection which may persist for a long time and lead to irreversible damage to the eye and eventual blindness.

MOLECULAR ASPECTS OF HERPES VIRUS INFECTION:
THE DEVELOPMENT OF LYTIC AND LATENT INFECTIONS

The initiation of a virus growth cycle within a cell creates a unique and threatening situation to the host. The virions are composed of a nucleic acid genome containing all the information essential for the duplication of the parental nucleic acid; but they lack the machinery needed for the manufacture of protein; and they depend on the cellular ribosomes and all the enzymes involved in this synthesis.

The virus nucleic acids transcribe mRNA molecules which can interact with the cell ribosomes and can direct the synthesis of viral proteins. Two major species of viral mRNA are transcribed from the viral genome: the "early" mRNA molecules which are copied from the parental DNA genomes; and "late" mRNA molecules which are transcribed from the DNA progeny. The herpes viruses are DNA viruses which replicate in the nucleus of the host cell. The fact that HS virus DNA molecules replicate only in the nucleus of the host cell points to their dependence on nuclear processes. This could lead to a) damage to the host cell chromosomes; b) inhibition of the synthesis of cellular DNA and RNA molecules; and c) integration of viral DNA genomes into the chromosomal DNA, resulting in cell transformation. Under certain conditions, HS virus is capable of seriously inhibiting host cell functions and initiating a lytic cycle in the cells. Under different conditions, a latent infection develops and the virus replicates only when induced. Under still other conditions the EB virus of the herpes group transforms human leukocytes and integrates its DNA genomes into the chromosomal DNA of the cells. The molecular processes which enable a herpes virus to lyse a cell, to become a latent virus or to transform a cell into a cancer cell are discussed below.

Molecular aspects of the lytic cycle of HS virus. 1) Initiation of infection; transcription of early mRNA: The viral genomes are rapidly transported after infection from the cytoplasm to the host cell nucleus as naked DNA molecules (25). In order for the viral DNA to function the early mRNA molecules must be transcribed. The nature of the DNA-dependent RNA polymerase which transcribes these viral mRNA molecules is not yet known. The early mRNA molecules must be released from the nucleus to the host cell cytoplasm, where they can interact with cellular ribosomes in order to be translated into viral proteins. The nature of these viral gene products is also not yet known, but it is clear that they are essential for the development of the virus growth cycle.

2) Replication of viral DNA: Viral DNA synthesis was studied following infection of synchronized BSC₁ cells with HS virus. It was found that viral DNA molecules are synthesized in the nuclei of the infected cells throughout the virus growth cycle. Synthesis of the viral DNA is carried out by an uncharacterized DNA-dependent DNA polymerase. Since treatment of infected cells with puromycin results in immediate decay of DNA-synthesizing activity, continuous protein synthesis appears to be required for the replication of the viral DNA. Thus, the enzymes which participate in the replication of HS virus DNA have a short half life (32) (Fig. 6).

3) Synthesis and transport of mRNA; the formation of polyribosomes: The late viral mRNA molecules are transcribed from the progeny of the viral DNA. Within 20 min viral mRNA molecules are transported from the nuclei to the cytoplasm (33) even in the absence of cellular protein synthesis. The viral RNA polymerase which transcribes the late mRNA molecules is more stable than the viral DNA polymerase, and continues to transcribe mRNA for 2 hr in the absence of protein synthesis before its activity decays (34). The viral mRNA molecules appear in the cytoplasm as free RNA molecules. Eventually, they interact with ribosomal subunits to form a mRNA-ribosome complex, the initial complex which leads to the formation of polyribosomes by the attachment of additional ribosomes to the mRNA molecules. However, the question of how a

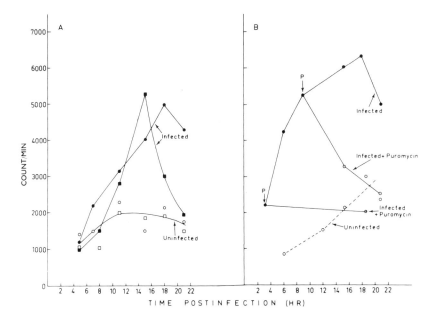

FIG. 6. Rate of DNA synthesis in cells infected with herpes virus. At 3-hr intervals, duplicate cultures of infected BSC_1 (green monkey kidney) cells were labeled with thymidine-C^{14} for 1 hr. The cells were then washed twice with phosphate buffered saline, dissolved in sodium dodecyl sulfate (SDS) buffer (Tris 0.005 M, NaCl 0.1 M, pH 7.3, SDS 0.5%), and the amount of radioactivity was determined. Uninfected cultures were similarly treated and analyzed. The results of two experiments are presented in Fig. 6A. The findings in a third experiment in which several infected cultures received 100 μg of puromycin per culture, at times indicated by "P", are shown in Fig. 6B. Each point in the curves represents the average value for two samples. DNA synthesis in infected cultures was markedly elevated and reached a maximum at 15 or 18 hr after infection. Puromycin, an inhibitor of protein synthesis, prevented any increase in DNA synthesis when added at 3 hr after infection. At 9 hr after infection, when a high level of DNA synthesis was already evident, puromycin caused a pronounced decline (———). Thus *de novo* protein synthesis is required for the synthesis of viral DNA.

cellular ribosome recognizes the viral mRNA and interacts with it is not yet resolved.

4) Synthesis of herpes virus structural proteins and their transport to the nuclei: Viral proteins are synthesized in the cytoplasm of the host cell whereas DNA replication occurs in the nuclei. Thus a mechanism must exist which permits the transport of the viral structural proteins to the nuclei. Several proteins (e.g., the glycoprotein for the outer virion

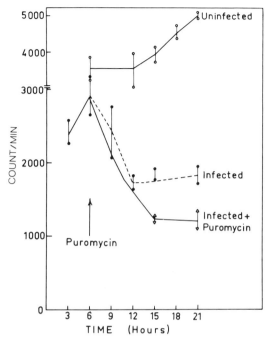

FIG. 7.   Rate of RNA synthesis in cells infected with HS virus.
Infected and uninfected BSC₁ (green monkey kidney) cells were labeled with H³-uridine for 60 min at 3-hr intervals. Some of the infected cultures received puromycin (20 μg/ml) 6 hr after infection. The cells were washed with phosphate buffered saline, dissolved in sodium dodecyl sulfate (SDS) buffer (Tris 0.005 M, NaCl 0.1 M, pH 7.3, SDS 0.5%), and the amount of radioactivity was determined. Uninfected cells exhibited a gradual increase in the rate of RNA synthesis, whereas cells infected with HS virus showed a decline. Inhibition of protein synthesis by puromycin (10 μg/ml) caused a still sharper drop in RNA synthesis. This could be due to inhibition of the synthesis of virus-induced RNA polymerase.

envelope) are retained in the cytoplasm but most of them are transported into the nuclei, where they function either as enzymes or as structural coat proteins for the assembly of the virions (34). The mechanism of protein transport is not yet fully understood.

5) Coating of herpes virus DNA; formation of virions: The virus structural proteins entering the infected nuclei form capsomeres which interact with each other to form empty capsids. The viral DNA molecules are incorporated into the latter and the nucleocapsids are then enveloped. Isolation of both incomplete and mature herpes virions on sucrose gradients made it possible to determine the kinetics of the formation of virions (35).

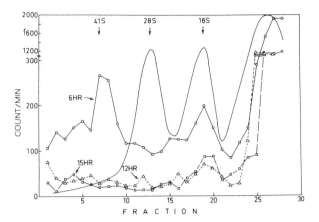

FIG. 8.   Effect of HS virus infection on cellular RNA synthesis.
BSC$_1$ (green monkey kidney) cells were pulsed for 20 min with H^3-uridine at 6, 12 and 15 hr after infection with HS virus. The cells were washed, dissolved in SDS buffer (see legend for Fig. 7), and centrifuged in 15 to 30% (w/w) sucrose gradients prepared in SDS buffer for 15 hr at 19,000 rev/min and 25 C, in the SW 25.1 rotor of the Beckman model L-2 ultracentrifuge. The OD$_{260nm}$ (———) was recorded automatically while each gradient was being collected in 27 fractions. The radioactivity in each fraction was then determined (other lines).
The 28 S and 18 S peaks indicate ribosomal RNA with sedimentation constants of 28 and 18 Svedberg units, respectively. At 6 hr after infection, the cells synthesized ribosomal precursor RNA (41 S) and heterogeneous RNA species, as occurs in normal uninfected cells. At 12 and 15 hr after infection, the synthesis of heterogeneous and ribosomal precursor RNA species was abolished and the synthesis of 18 S RNA molecules was reduced.

Analysis of the proteins in the complete and incomplete particles suggested the following sequence of interaction between the different proteins: Proteins VIII and II compose the empty capsid. The internal proteins (VII and VI) interact with the DNA and organize it into a globular structure which can be incorporated into the capsid. The subsequent stages of the formation of the HS virions are a) interaction inside the infected nuclei of the nucleocapsids with membranes which contain a virus-specific glycoprotein (protein IV); b) interaction of the partially enveloped nucleocapsids with the nuclear membrane, which also contains viral glycoprotein (protein V); and c) release of the virion into the host cell cytoplasm, where it obtains the last and the largest envelope, containing a virus-specific glycoprotein (protein III). The lipid moiety of the membrane is of cellular origin, while the glycoproteins are specified by the virus. The mature herpes virions are then released from the cytoplasm of the infected cell and can infect new host cells.

Effect of herpes virus infection on the host cell. When HS virus infects growing cells which synthesize DNA, the rate of the cellular DNA synthesis rapidly declines, while viral DNA synthesis gradually increases (36). Infection with HS virus can also cause breakage of chromosomal DNA (37). The mechanism responsible for the inhibition of the synthesis of cellular DNA has not yet been determined.

In addition, infection with HS virus completely inhibits the synthesis of the cellular ribosomal precursor RNA (34) (Fig. 7). Thus, the infected cells cannot synthesize new ribosomal subunits and the translation of the cell mRNA molecules is therefore inhibited. The infected cells are able to synthesize transfer RNA (Fig. 8). Due to the virus infection, the nucleoli of the infected cells disaggregate and disappear, by means not yet recognized.

As a result of the inhibitory effects on the host DNA and RNA synthesis, the ability of the infected cells to synthesize proteins rapidly declines, while the synthesis of viral proteins gradually increases.

Thus, under conditions which permit the expression of all the viral genes, the functions of the host cell are inhibited and the cell is finally destroyed in the course of the lytic virus cycle.

Under different cellular conditions, the expression of only part of the viral genes is permitted by the host cell. Such a situation prevents the synthesis of virions, enables the infected cell to exist and permits the virus to become latent.

Molecular events in latent infection with HS virus. HS virus can exist in infected tissue without any sign until its replication is induced as a result of physiological changes in the host organism (38, 39). Furthermore, HS virus can infect certain cells, for example nerve cells (even traveling along them), but remains entirely latent. Lytic virus infections can erupt in adjacent, susceptible cells, as in tissue cells near nerve endings (38). These observations indicate that the viral DNA genome may be present in nerve cells for some time without being able to replicate. Obviously the expression of viral genes can occur only in permissive cells. What is the molecular basis of this control over viral expression? It has become evident in recent years that the replication of herpes virus can be prevented in cells incubated in medium deficient in arginine (40). It is also possible that the host cell may control the expression of viral genes by preventing the transcription of the viral early mRNA.

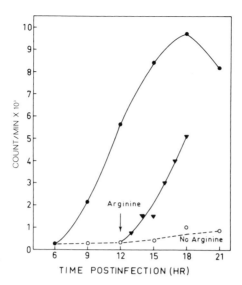

FIG. 9. Effect of arginine deprivation on HS virus replication and the reversal of the deficiency effect.

BSC$_1$ (green monkey kidney) cell cultures infected with herpes virus in the presence or absence of arginine were each labeled with H^3- thymidine. Samples were withdrawn at different times. The cells were scraped into reticulocyte standard buffer (10^{-2} M KCl, 10^{-2} M Tris, pH 7.4, 1.5 × 10^{-3} M Mg^{++}) and disrupted ultrasonically. The amount of radioactive DNA present before and after treatment with deoxyribonuclease (DNase) was determined.

Incubation of HS virus from infected cell suspensions with DNase for 30 min at 37 C in the presence of 10^{-2} M Mg^{++} results in the degradation of all exposed DNA, leaving the encapsidated viral DNA intact. At 12 hr after infection the arginine in some cultures was restored to normal concentration in Eagle's medium and samples were taken every hour.

HS virus was able to replicate in complete medium (●———●), or, when arginine was replaced, in deficient medium. However, in the absence of arginine no radioactively labeled virus could be demonstrated.

The role of these processes in the development of a latent infection remains to be studied.

1) Arginine deprivation; inhibition of HS virus replication: Arginine deprivation affects HS virus replication in that although viral DNA is synthesized in the deprived cells, coating of the DNA is prevented and virions are not formed. Viral antigens and viral structural proteins are synthesized in the deprived cells, but at a low rate, and they do not assemble into capsids. Addition of arginine to the deprived cultures results

in the formation of virions (Fig. 9) which contain viral proteins synthesized in the cells in the absence of arginine (41).

It is possible that in the absence of arginine the host cell is unable to provide the herpes virus with a cellular function necessary for virion formation or that arginine is needed for viral protein synthesis itself. Although the effect of arginine deprivation on virion formation is recognized the effect on the host cell has not yet been determined. In another herpes virus-host model (EB virus and Burkitt's lymphoblasts), arginine deprivation primarily affects the host and causes a regulatory change in the lympoblasts.

2) Herpes virus latency due to lack of early transcription: The mechanism of early viral mRNA transcription after HS virus infection is not yet known and the possibility exists that a cellular DNA-dependent RNA polymerase is required for this process. If a cellular enzyme indeed participates in the early transcription as demonstrated in bacteriophage T4 infections (42), the presence or absence of the cellular RNA polymerase may directly control the course of infection with herpes virus. To date, three cellular DNA-dependent RNA polymerases have been isolated from mammalian cells (20): a nucleolar RNA polymerase which transcribes the ribosomal precursor RNA molecules, and two RNA polymerases in the nucleoplasm. If herpes virions enter a cell which lacks the polymerase capable of transcribing early viral mRNA, the viral DNA genomes may possibly remain in a latent form. Changes in the cells, such as those due to stimulation by hormones, which lead to the synthesis of cellular RNA polymerase, would then also lead to the transcription of the latent viral DNA genomes and to the development of a lytic infection. The cellular enzyme necessary for early viral DNA transcription may be generally lacking in nerve cells, but may be present in the cells near the nerve endings which permit virus replication.

CELL-DNA VIRUS INTERACTION LEADING TO NEOPLASTIC
CELL TRANSFORMATION AND THE DEVELOPMENT OF CANCER

Viruses and cancer. Studies on DNA viruses which transform cells *in vitro* have demonstrated a new type of host-virus interaction. These DNA viruses (43), as well as some RNA viruses (13), change the regulatory processes in the infected host in such a manner as to bestow on the clone the ability to grow indefinitely. Whereas RNA tumor viruses can multiply in the transformed cell the DNA tumor viruses are unable to replicate.

Studies on the interaction of tumorogenic DNA viruses with host cells have shown the following: a) In order to fix the transformed state, the infected cell must replicate its DNA and divide. b) Viral DNA (as in the case of SV_{40} polyoma and adenoviruses) is integrated into the host cell DNA at the rate of about 25 copies of the viral DNA per cellular genome. c) Only part of the viral DNA is transcribed when it is integrated into the host cell DNA (44). The cellular mRNA molecules contain information for the early viral functions. d) Treatment of the transformed cells with mitomycin C results in the release of viral DNA genomes from their integrated state (45). The released viral DNA genomes can replicate and transcribe late mRNA molecules, which are translated into structural proteins, leading to the formation of virions. e) The viral genomes can be released from their integrated state in the transformed cells by fusing the cancer cells with normal ones.

Such a series of events may take place in human Burkitt lymphoblasts, which have been found to contain an agent of the herpes group, designated EB virus, which was isolated from the EB_3 cell-line of African human lymphoma (46). Similarly, herpes viruses have been found to be associated with renal tumors of the leopard frog (Lucké virus) and with tumors of chickens (Marek's disease virus). Since EB virus is associated with human cancer, it is of obvious importance to investigate the processes which lead to the development of tumors in human beings and to study the relations between the human lymphoblast and its associated herpes virus.

EB virus and human lymphoma. 1) Presence of EB virus antigens and viral DNA in human cancer cells: Electron miscroscopic studies of lymphoblasts isolated from African lymphoma patients and cultivated *in vitro* (46) have disclosed the presence of herpes virus particles in the nuclei of 70% of the cells. The presence of the virions in these cells is associated with the occurrence of virus-controlled antigens which react with antibodies found in the blood of the lymphoma patients (47, 48). When lymphoblasts which did not have EB virions were cloned, all clones were found to include cells which contained these virions. It follows that EB virus DNA may be present in each lymphoblast.

2) Characterization of EB virus: Analyses of EB virions, purified on sucrose gradients, disclosed that the virions contain DNA molecules with a molecular weight of 100×10^6 daltons and a density of 1.719 ± 0.001 g/cm^3. The virions have a protein coat composed of nine major proteins which resemble the coat proteins of HS virus in their electro-

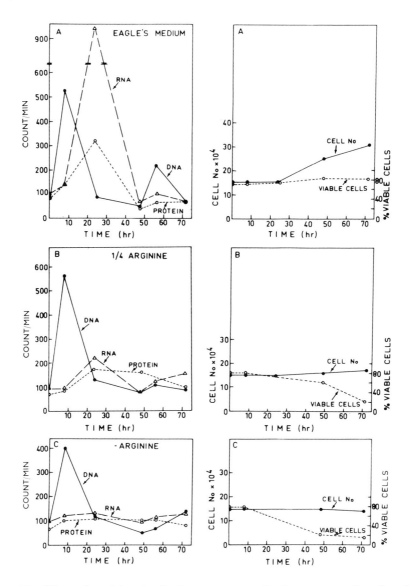

FIG. 10. Effect of arginine deprivation on macromolecular processes in cultured Burkitt lymphoblasts.

EB₃ Burkitt lymphoblasts, obtained from an African lymphoma patient, were incubated in complete Eagle's medium (A), medium containing a quarter of the regular arginine concentration (B) or medium without arginine (C). After various time intervals the rates of RNA, DNA and protein synthesis were determined by labeling samples of each cell preparation for 1 hr with H³-uridine, H³-thymidine.

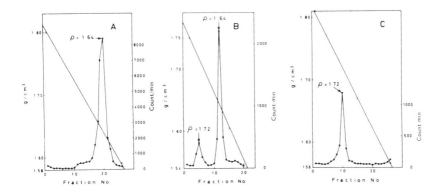

FIG. 11. Characterization of the DNA synthesized in arginine-deprived Burkitt lymphoblasts.

EB$_3$ cells were resuspended in fresh Eagle's medium (A), or in Eagle's medium without arginine (B), and incubated for hr at 37 C in the presence of H^3-thymidine. The cells were harvested and resuspended in phosphate buffer, pH 6.4. The nuclei were obtained by homogenization of the cells in a Dounce glass homogenizer, incubated overnight at 37 C with pronase (500 μg) in the presence of 1% (w/w) sodium deoxycholate and 1% (w/w) sodium dodecyl sulfate. Cesium chloride crystals were added to each preparation to an initial density of 1.69 g/cm^3. The gradients were centrifuged for 48 hr in the SW 39 rotor of a Beckman model L-2 preparative ultracentrifuge. Samples were collected and the density and radioactivity were determined.

All the DNA molecules synthesized in EB$_3$ cells suspended in complete Eagle's medium had a density of 1.64 g/cm^3 (A). The low density (1.64 g/ml) is due to protein contamination of the isolated cell DNA. When conditions for deproteinization are improved, the density of the DNA becomes 1.696 g/cm^3. In arginine-deprived cells (B), most of the DNA also had a density of 1.64 g/cm^3 which corresponds to cellular DNA, while about 20% of the radioactive DNA molecules had a density of 1.72 g/cm^3, similar to the density of HS virus DNA (C). ρ = density.

---

or C^{14}-protein hydrolysate, respectively (left panel). In addition, the cells were stained with trypan blue at different time intervals and the total number of cells as well as the number of viable cells was determined (right panel).

Incubation of EB$_3$ cells in arginine-free medium resulted in a marked inhibition of the synthesis of both RNA and proteins, and in abolition of the G2 phase of the cell growth cycle (C) in contrast to cells in complete medium (A). The presence of a quarter of the regular concentration of arginine did not restore the ability of the cells to synthesize RNA and proteins. The synthesis of DNA was reduced to only about 50% (B, C) as compared to control cells (A), and a distinct S period was still evident. Cell growth was inhibited when arginine was partially (B) or completely (C) removed and the number of living cells gradually declined.

phoretic mobilities (49). However, the two agents differ in antigenicity.

3) Induction of EB virus replication in lymphoblasts by arginine deprivation: That EB virus DNA may exist in the lymphoblasts which do not show virions was suggested by experiments in which the cells were incubated in an arginine-deficient medium. Under these conditions viral capsid antigens appear in up to 75% of the cells (50). Analysis of the effect of arginine deprivation on cultured EB₃ Burkitt lymphoblasts (Fig. 10) demonstrated that the deprived cells are capable of synthesizing DNA during the S phase but that the synthesis of RNA and proteins during the G2 phase is completely prevented (51). Analysis by CsCl density centrifugation of the DNA synthesized in the arginine-deprived lymphoblasts demonstrated that in addition to cell DNA, EB virus DNA molecules are synthesized in the nuclei (Fig. 11). The amount of EB virus DNA gradually increases during the initial 20 hr after arginine deprivation. After this, viral DNA is able to code for the synthesis of the viral coat proteins and mature virions are formed four days later.

These studies indicate that a) The EB virus DNA molecules may be integrated in the DNA of the lymphoblast. b) When a change occurs in the cell which permits breakage of cellular DNA the viral genomes are released. c) The released viral genomes can replicate and code for the synthesis of late viral functions. It is possible that arginine deprivation induces the synthesis of late viral functions. It is also possible that arginine deprivation induces the synthesis of an excision enzyme which permits the release of viral genomes from the integrated state (52). Further studies have indeed shown that the viral DNA molecules are integrated into the host cell DNA; six copies of the viral DNA in each lymphoblast (52).

Transformation of human lymphocytes. The demonstration that EB virus DNA may be intimately associated with chromosomal DNA in the lymphoblast suggests that the EB virus may indeed be responsible for the transformation of the lymphocyte; and it was found that incubation of human lymphocytes from peripheral blood with a crude suspension of EB virus (53) gives rise to the appearance of transformed cells resembling Burkitt lymphoblasts. Infectious mononucleosis is the outcome of an *in vivo* infection of white blood cells with EB virus (54). These studies point to a unique type of cell-virus relationship. Upon infecting a lymphocyte, EB virus is able to change the control mechanism of the cell and to cause a permanent change manifested by abnormal growth properties. The infected cell is capable of preventing the herpes virus from expressing its late functions and the viral DNA is integrated into DNA of the host cell. The molecular processes involved in the transformation of a normal human cell into a cancer cell await description.

CONCLUSIONS

Analysis of the interaction of a mammalian cell with an obligate parasite profoundly involves both the host and the parasite. Understanding of the nature of such interactions at the molecular level therefore requires detailed studies of the physiology of the cells as well as of the parasites. Although such studies are still largely initial, it is already possible to conclude that viral parasites, upon entry into a host, trigger both cellular- and parasite-specific processes which determine the fate of the interaction. Events in cells infected with a prokaryotic parasite like the trachoma agent differ markedly from those which occur as a result of a virus infection, as in the case of HS virus. Viruses which function inside the cell as naked DNA molecules maintain themselves by utilizing cellular molecular processes. Depending on the host cell which they invade they are subjected to processes which may affect the ability of the viral genome to function; and to a change from a cell-destructive lytic cycle to a situation in which the cell controls the viral genome and causes virus latency.

The most intriguing process in host-virus interaction is the neoplastic transformation of a cell by a viral agent. In such circumstances viral DNA is integrated into the host DNA, and the cell, after one division, becomes a cancer cell. Understanding of the processes which allow different viruses to be integrated into host chromosomal DNA, knowledge of the exact location of the viral DNA molecules in the cellular genome and clarification of the processes which enable the infected-transformed cell to synthesize its DNA and to replicate, are likely to shed light on the molecular mechanisms of carcinogenesis. It is not impossible that such insights may eventually lead to the development of new tools to reverse or inhibit these processes, and thereby to the control of virus-induced human neoplasia.

The experimental work from the author's laboratory discussed in this paper was carried out in collaboration with I. Sarov, Z. Zakay-Rones, E. Hochberg, H. Loker, B. Gutter, H. Dym, Y. Asher, J. Levitt-Hadar, U. Olshevsky and A. Weinberg, whom the author wishes to thank. The capable technical assistance of N. Himmel, K. Press, M. Dreifus and E. Eynav is greatly appreciated.

Supported by grants from the National Institutes of Health, Bethesda, Md, USA; from the World Health Organization, Geneva, Switzerland; from the Leukemia Research Foundation, Inc, Chicago, Ill and from Gruppo Lepetit, Milan, Italy.

REFERENCES

1. BERNKOPF H, MASHIAH P and BECKER Y. Correlation between morphological and biochemical changes and the appearance of infectivity in FL cell cultures infected with trachoma agent. *Ann NY Acad Sci* **98**: 62–81, 1962.
2. OSSOWSKI L, BECKER Y and BERNKOPF H. Amino acid requirements of trachoma strains and other agents of the PLT group in cell culture. *Isr J Med Sci* **1**: 186–193, 1965.
3. SAROV I and BECKER Y. Trachoma agent DNA. *J Mol Biol* **42**: 581–589, 1969.
4. SAROV I and BECKER Y. RNA in the elementary bodies of trachoma agent. *Nature (Lond)* **217**: 849–852, 1968.
4a. GUTTER B and BECKER Y. Synthesis and maturation of trachoma agent ribosomal RNA. *J Mol Biol* **66**: 239, 1972.
5. SAROV I and BECKER Y. DNA dependent RNA polymerase in the trachoma elementary bodies, in: Nichole RL (Ed), "Trachoma and related disorders caused by chlamydial agents." Amsterdam, Excerpta Medica, 1971, pp 27–33.
6. SAROV I and BECKER Y. DNA dependent RNA polymerase activity in purified trachoma elementary bodies: the effect of NaCl on RNA transcription. *J Bacteriol* **107**: 593–599, 1971.
7. BECKER Y and ZAKAY-RONES Z. Rifampicin—a new antitrachoma drug. *Nature (Lond)* **222**: 851–853, 1969.
8. BECKER Y. Cure and eradication of trachoma agent by the antibiotic rifampicin. Proc 21st Int Congr Ophthalmology, Mexico City, March 1970. Amsterdam, Excerpta Medica, 1971, pp 1921–1926.
9. BECKER Y, LOKER H, SAROV I, ASHER Y, GUTTER B and ZAKAY-RONES Z. The molecular biology of trachoma agent, in Nichole RL (Ed), "Trachoma and related disorders caused by chlamydial agents." Amsterdam, Excerpta Medica, 1971, pp 13–26.
10. MOULDER JW, The relation of the psittacosis group (Chlamydiae) to bacteria and viruses. *Annu Rev Microbiol* **20**: 107–130, 1966.
11. KATES JR and MCAUSLAN BR. Poxvirus DNA-dependent RNA polymerase. *Proc Natl Acad Sci USA* **58**: 134–141, 1967.
12. BALTIMORE, D. Viral RNA-dependent DNA polymerase. *Nature (Lond)* **226**: 1209–1211, 1970.
13. TEMIN H and MIZUTANI S. RNA-dependent DNA polymerase in virions of Rous sarcoma virus. *Nature (Lond)* **226**: 1211, 1970.
14. WILDY P and WATSON DH. Electron microscopic studies on the architecture of animal viruses. *Cold Spr Harb Symp Quant Biol* **27**: 25–47, 1962.
15. NII S, MORGAN C and ROSE HM. Electron microscopy of herpes simplex virus. II. Sequence of development. *J Virol* **2**: 517–536, 1968.
16. BECKER Y, DYM H and SAROV I. Herpes simplex virus DNA. *Virology* **36**: 184–192, 1968.
17. OLSHEVSKY U and BECKER Y. Herpes simplex virus structural proteins. *Virology* **40**: 948–960, 1970.
18. ASHER Y, HELLER M and BECKER Y. Incorporation of lipids into herpes simplex virions. *J Gen Virol* **4**: 65–76, 1969.
19. DARNELL JE. Ribonucleic acids from animal cells. *Bacteriol Rev* **32**: 262–290, 1968.
20. ROEDER RG and RUTTER WJ. Multiple forms of DNA-dependent RNA polymerase in eukaryotic organisms. *Nature (Lond)* **224**: 234–237, 1970.
21. JOKLIK WK and BECKER Y. Studies on the genesis of polyribosomes. II. The *J Mol Biol* **13**: 499–510, 1965.
    association of nascent messenger RNA with the 40 S subribosomal particles.
22. RICH, A PENMAN S, BECKER Y and DARNELL, JE. Polyribosomes: size in normal and polio infected HeLa cells. *Science* **142**: 1658–1663, 1963.
23. LENGYEL P and SÖLL D. Mechanism of protein biosynthesis. *Bacteriol Rev* **33**: 264–301, 1969.

24. BECKER Y, HOCHBERG E and ZAKAY-RONES Z. Interaction of trachoma elementary bodies with host cells. *Isr J Med Sci* **5**: 121–124, 1969.
25. HOCHBERG E and BECKER Y. The adsorption, penetration and uncoating of herpes simplex virus in BSC_1 cells. *J Gen Virol* **2**: 231–241, 1968.
26. BERNKOPF H, MASHIAH P and BECKER Y. Correlation between morphological and biochemical changes and the appearance of infectivity in FL cell cultures infected with trachoma agent. *Ann NY Acad Sci* **98**: 62–81, 1962.
27. COLBY C and CHAMBERLIN MI. The specificity of interferon induction in chick embryo cells by helical RNA. *Proc Natl Acad Sci USA* **63**: 160–167, 1969.
28. MERIGNAN T and HANNAH L. Characteristics of interferon induced *in vitro* and *in vivo* by a TRIC agent. *Proc Soc Exp Biol Med* **122**: 421–424, 1966.
29. DIANZANI F, BUCKLER CE and BARON S. Effect of cycloheximide on the antiviral action of interferon. *Proc Soc Exp Biol Med* **130**: 519–523, 1969.
30. GUTTER B, SAROV I and BECKER Y. Studies on trachoma agent DNA-dependent RNA polymerase. *Isr J Chem* **8**: 125, 1970.
31. ALEXANDER JJ. Separation of protein synthesis in meningopneumonitis agent from that in the L cells by differential susceptibility to cycloheximide. *J Bacteriol* **95**: 327–332, 1968.
32. LEVITT-HADAR J. Molecular events in the replication of a nuclear DNA virus: Herpes simplex virus. PhD thesis, Hebrew University of Jerusalem, 1970.
33. WAGNER EK and ROIZMAN B. RNA synthesis in cells infected with herpes simplex virus. II. Evidence that a class of viral mRNA is derived from a high molecular weight precursor synthesized in the nucleus. *Proc Natl Acad Sci USA* **64**: 626–633, 1969.
34. KIEF E, ROIZMAN B and BECKER Y. Synthesis, transport and function of herpes simplex virus messenger RNA in the presence of puromycin. *Bacteriol Proc* 1971, p 219.
35. OLSHEVSKY U, LEVITT J and BECKER Y. Studies on the synthesis of herpes simplex virions. *Virology* **33**: 324–334, 1967.
36. ROIZMAN B and ROANE PR. The multiplication of herpes simplex virus. II. The relation between protein synthesis and the duplication of viral DNA in infected HEp-2 cells. *Virology* **22**: 262–269, 1964.
37. HAMPAR BH and ALLISON SA. Cellular alterations in the MCH line of Chinese hamster cells following infection with herpes simplex virus. *Proc Natl Acad Sci USA* **49**: 474–480, 1963.
38. SCOTT TFMcN and KOKUMARO T. Herpes virus hominis (virus of herpes simplex). *Bacteriol Rev* **28**: 458–471, 1964.
39. KAPLAN AS and BEN-PORAT T. Metabolism of animal cells infected with nuclear DNA viruses. *Annu Rev Microbiol* **22**: 427–450, 1968.
40. BECKER Y, OLSHEVSKY U and LEVITT J. The role of arginine in the replication of herpes virus. *J Gen Virol* **1**: 471–478, 1967.
41. OLSHEVSKY U and BECKER Y. Synthesis of herpes simplex virus structural proteins in arginine deprived cells. *Nature (Lond)* **226**: 851–853, 1970.
42. GEIDUSCHEK EP and SKLAR J. Role of host RNA polymerase in phage development. *Nature (Lond)* **221**: 833, 1969.
43. BLACK PH. The oncogenic DNA viruses: A review of *in vitro* transformation studies. *Annu Rev Microbiol* **22**: 391–426, 1968.
44. DULBECCO R. The state of the DNA of polyoma virus and SV_{40} in transformed cells. *Cold Spr Harb Symp Quant Biol* **33**: 777–783, 1968.
45. BURNS WH and BLACK PH. Analysis of SV_{40}-induced transformation of hamster kidney tissue *in vitro*. *Virology* **39**: 625–634, 1969.
46. EPSTEIN MA and BARR YM. Virus particles in cultured lymphoblasts from Burkitt's lymphoma. *Lancet* **i**: 702–703, 1964.
47. HENLE G and HENLE W. Immunofluorescence in cells derived from Burkitt's lymphoma. *J Bacteriol* **91**: 1248–1256, 1966.
48. KLEIN G, CLIFFORD P, KLEIN E, SMITH RT, MINOWADA J, KOURILSKY FM and BURCHENAL JH. Membrane immunofluorescence reactions of Burkitt

lymphoma cells from biopsy specimens and tissue cultures. *J Natl Cancer Inst*
39: 1027–1044, 1967.
49. WEINBERG A and BECKER Y. Studies on EB virus of Burkitt's lymphoblasts.
Virology **39**: 312–321, 1969.
50. HENLE W and HENLE G. Effect of arginine-deficient media on the herpes-
type virus associated with cultured Burkitt tumor cells. *J Virol* **2**: 182–191,
1968.
51. WEINBERG A and BECKER Y. Effect of arginine deprivation on macromolecular processes in Burkitt's lymphoblasts. *Exp Cell Res* **60**: 470–474, 1970.
52. ZUR HAUSEN H and SCHULTE-HOLTHAUSEN H. Presence of EB virus nucleic
acid homology in a "virus free" line of Burkitt tumor cells. *Nature (Lond)*
227: 245–248, 1970.
53. POPE JH, HORNE MR and SCOTT W. Transformation of foetal human leukocytes *in vitro* by filtrates of a human leukaemic cell line containing herpes-
like virus. *Int J Cancer* **3**: 857–866, 1968.
54. HENLE G, HENLE W and DIEHL V. Relation of Burkitt's tumor-associated
herpes type virus to infectious mononucleosis. *Proc Natl Acad Sci USA* **59**:
94–101, 1968.

HOST-PARASITE RELATIONSHIPS IN DISEASES CAUSED BY GROUP A STREPTOCOCCI

ISAAC GINSBURG

Laboratory for Microbiology and Immunology, Faculty of Dental Medicine,
Hebrew University–Alpha Omega Research and Postgraduate Center,
Jerusalem, Israel

A) INTRODUCTION AND BACKGROUND

The role played by group A hemolytic streptococci in the pathogenesis of human disease has attracted the interest of numerous investigators since the beginning of the century. This interest stems from the fact that these microorganisms are responsible for causing many different forms of acute and highly contagious diseases, the most common of which are tonsillitis, pharyngitis and scarlet fever. Moreover, a certain percentage of human beings suffering from such diseases develop specific, chronic and sometimes crippling sequelae such as rheumatic fever, acute glomerulonephritis and arthritis a few weeks after the onset of infection. These secondary pathological processes are inflammatory and nonsuppurative, and involve the connective tissue of the heart muscle and heart valves, the glomeruli of the kidneys and the synovial membrane of the joints. These complications tend to be chronic or recurrent, and frequently lead to serious cardiac and kidney disorders.

Although numerous epidemiological and clinical studies have shown a definite relationship between a preceding infection with strains of group A streptococci and the appearance of such sequelae, the mechanisms which lead to their development are still not fully understood.

Since human beings are the only animal species which suffer from natural infections with group A streptococci, and since streptococci cannot usually be isolated from the lesions characteristic of the chronic complications, Koch's postulates can at best incriminate these microorganisms only in the etiology of the acute infections, but not in their subsequent complications. Many attempts have been made to duplicate rheumatic fever, nephritis and arthritis in experimental animals. These have involved the inoculation of streptococcal strains, freshly isolated from patients who later developed one or more of the sequelae, into a variety of laboratory and domestic animals by various routes. As a rule, however, the tissue lesions which develop in some of these animals bear little resemblance to the human lesions, and no true duplication of a disease syndrome similar to that seen in human beings has been reported.

Two major theories have been proposed to explain the nature of the poststreptococcal diseases. One theory holds that the chronic lesions represent the consequences of the direct toxic effects of some streptococcal products on the tissues. The second theory suggests that immunopathological phenomena develop in patients who have become sensitized to one or more of the streptococcal products. This suggestion is based on the analogy between the pathological alterations seen in poststreptococcal diseases and the experimental lesions which develop in animals repeatedly exposed to certain foreign proteins. The immunological approach is also attractive since it is well established that two to three weeks must usually elapse between the onset of acute infections with streptococci and the appearance of the complications. This is the period of time needed to develop an adequate immune response.

These two hypotheses are not, of course, mutually exclusive. Although no unified theory has been advanced which adequately explains the nature of the various poststreptococcal complications, a combination of both views may fit many, if not all, the features characteristic of these sequelae. The purpose of this essay is to attempt an integrative analysis of the mechanisms of both acute and chronic human disease initiated by streptococci on the basis of observations of the reaction of experimental hosts to these bacteria and their products.

B) BIOLOGICAL PROPERTIES OF GROUP A STREPTOCOCCI

Definition of the major biological properties of the streptococcus (1) is obviously a prerequisite to an attempt to understand the nature of its association with a host.

The hemolytic streptococcus is a fastidious, gram-positive, parasitic bacterium which, during long association with the human host, has lost the ability to synthesize many proteins and enzymes, and which is therefore dependent on the host for many of its metabolic building blocks. Thus, nutritional requirements for at least 13 amino acids, four vitamins, a number of purines and pyrimidines, as well as for some ready-made peptides have been demonstrated (2). It would stand to reason that the streptococcus has developed numerous extracellular agents capable of attacking and degrading cells and tissues for the purpose of securing growth factors as compensation for its loss of synthetic capacity. The organism derives its energy by splitting glucose and other fermentable sugars to lactic acid (1), and one of the most prominent characteristics of the streptococcal microenvironment is its high acidity. This property may have far-reaching implications in the pathogenesis of tissue injury.

The streptococcus possesses a rigid cell wall, composed of a branched polymer of N-acetylglucosamine (NAGA) and rhamnose, which is linked to NAGA-muranic acid, the branches of which are interconnected by a tetrapeptide. The principal serologically reactive component of the streptococcal cell wall is the NAGA and rhamnose polymer, known as C-polysaccharide (3, 4). This component is haptenic and confers upon the organism its group specificity. The rigid cell wall very seldom undergoes the autolysis frequently seen in many other bacterial species (5). The high resistance of the cell wall to the digestive effects of the host enzymes allows the streptococcus to persist in the tissues long after it has been killed by phagocytic cells (6). Thus, some of the most severe tissue alterations seen after streptococcal penetration result from the interactions of the cell wall components with different elements of connective tissue (6, 7). Many streptococcal strains secrete a superficial hyaluronic acid capsule (8) which, together with the type specific M-protein antigen (9), impedes phagocytosis and thus constitutes the main virulence factor of group A streptococci (10, 11).

The streptococcus localizes selectively in the upper respiratory tract, where it usually finds refuge in the deep crypts of the tonsils. In the absence of tonsils, the streptococcus may invade the deep cervical lymph glands and the deep fasciae of the neck and there cause cellulitis and initiate septicemia. On the other hand, certain streptococcal strains are primarily associated with skin infections (impetigo) (12).

At least 60 different serological types of group A streptococci have been recognized. Classification is based on the presence in the cell wall of the type-specific M-protein antigen (9). It is because of this antigenic heterogeneity that immunity to group A streptococci is type-specific. Consequently, a new streptococcal type appearing in a community often meets with only very low host resistance, and high incidence levels and considerable morbidity may therefore characterize epidemic streptococcal disease. The frequent passage of streptococci in the tissues of human beings, as in laboratory animals, is believed to enhance their virulence. While the majority of group A types may be associated with the development of rheumatic fever (rheumatogenic strains), only a very few strains have been implicated as nephritogenic.

Many forms of disease caused by streptococci have been defined. The most common ones are tonsillitis, pharyngitis, cervical adenitis, scarlet fever, puerperal fever, erysipelas and impetigo. The clinical manifestations of streptococcal infections sometimes depend on the state of immunity of the host. These diseases may appear in epidemic form in overcrowded populations such as schools, dormitories and army barracks. If adequate antibiotic treatment is not promptly given, septicemia and even death may ensue. Inadequate treatment may also lead to the development of crippling sequelae, the results of complex interactions between the streptococcus and the host.

C) HOW EXTRACELLULAR TOXINS OF STREPTOCOCCI COUNTERACT HOST RESPONSES

The streptococcus, which usually multiplies very rapidly in the rich environment of the host, produces large amounts of lactic acid and other metabolites of low molecular weight, as well as many antigenic macromolecular materials (13, 14). At least 25 different antigenic substances have been identified in culture supernates of group A streptococci (13, 14) by the use of immunoelectrophoretic techniques employing the γ-globulin fractions of sera from human beings convalescing from streptococcal infection. The presence of so many antistreptococcal antibodies in patients indicates that these antigenic substances are indeed elaborated *in vivo* (13, 14).

Very little is known about the mechanisms by which the streptococcus releases such macromolecules. It is believed, however, that these substances are end products of metabolism, and that autolytic processes are probably not involved in their secretion.

The streptococcus can be classified between the categories of toxigenic, noninvasive microorganisms (e.g., *Corynebacterium diphtheriae, Clostridium tetani*) and of invasive ones (e.g., pneumococci, anthrax bacilli). Although no specific streptococcal exoproduct has been incriminated as a unique "virulence factor," several of the streptococcal toxins (hemolysins, proteases) bring about partial collapse of host defenses.

Most of the exoproducts of the streptococci are elaborated during

TABLE 1. *Group A streptococcal components (extracellular products)*

	Selected references		Selected references
Proteinase precursor	38	SLS	15, 18, 23–25, 27
Proteinase (active)	39–43	Cell SF	116–119
NAD-glycohydrolase	62–66	SK	44, 45, 48, 51, 53
Hyaluronidase	54, 56	Nephrotoxin	85–91
Deoxyribonuclease A, B. C, D	58, 60	Mitogen	145, 146
Ribonuclease	58	Erythrogenic toxin	27, 68–70
SLO	15–17, 23–25, 27	Cardiohepatic toxins	76–78

TABLE 2. *Group A streptococcal components (cell wall and intracellular components)*

	Selected references
Hyaluronic acid	94–96
M-protein	92–94
T-protein ⎫ R-protein ⎬	3, 4
C-polysaccharide	3, 4, 106, 107
Mucopeptide	3, 4, 106, 107
Protoplast membrane	139, 140
Intracellular hemolysin	18
Intracellular SLO ⎫ Intracellular SLS ⎬	18
CBH (cell-bound SLS)	18
Nucleoprotein	1
Cross-reactive antigens (with kidney, cardiac muscle and valves, connective tissue)	121–124
Lipoproteinase Phosphatase Esterase N-acetylglucosaminidase α-amylase β-glucuronidase Dehydrogenases Adenosine triphosphatase	1, 13, 27, 67, 104

the logarithmic phase of growth. The majority are proteins, but small amounts of teichoic acids and some polysaccharides can also be found in culture supernates. Of the many streptococcal products released during growth, at least 13 are enzymes (Tables 1 and 2).

Since the environment of the streptococcal organism *in vivo* is probably rich in its exoproducts, it is conceivable that a phagocytic cell approaching such a site has to traverse a micro-milieu which contains many of these products. Thus, the consequences of the leukocytic migration resulting from accumulation of chemotactic factors depend to a considerable extent on whether the streptococcus can modify and cripple the leukocytes. Delay in the phagocytosis of the streptococci would allow the accumulation of more toxic factors, which might affect not only the immediate environment but might diffuse to other tissues and organs to cause widespread tissue damage (see below).

1) *Hemolysins and leukocidins.* Streptococci have long been known to hemolyse red blood cells of many animal species. Edgar Todd (15) was the first to demonstrate that streptococci isolated from human beings could elaborate two distinct extracellular hemolytic substances, which he named oxygen-labile Streptolysin O (SLO) to indicate its sensitivity to oxygen, and oxygen-stable Streptolysin S (SLS) to indicate its stability to oxygen and its high solubility in serum. While SLO can be found in supernates of streptococcal cultures grown in ordinary or in defined media (16, 17), SLS has, as a rule, been found only in cultures grown in the presence of serum (15, 18). Most of the β-hemolysis seen around colonies of group A streptococci cultivated on blood agar is considered to be due to SLS (18).

SLO is a protein with a mol wt of approximately 65,000, which can be reversibly oxidized and reduced. Its activity is associated with the reduced form (16).

SLS, according to the older definition, is that hemolytic substance elaborated by streptococci which is "extracted" from the bacterial cells by serum protein. Studies on the nature of SLS have been complicated by the fact that exhaustively washed streptococcal cells can hemolyse red blood cells, but that no hemolytic substance can be detected in the supernatant fluid of such cell suspensions. Hemolysis by washed streptococci was found to be due to a cell-bound hemolysin (CBH) (18, 19). Upon the addition of serum proteins, CBH is released from the streptococci to become complexed with serum proteins, and is thus recognized as SLS (19). Other materials, such as RNA, Tween and Triton can also serve as "extractors" (18). SLS is thought to be a complex between a specific hemolytic moiety, a peptide with a mol wt of 10,000 (20) synthesized by the streptococcus, and a nonspecific carrier (18, 19). The hemolytic moiety may be transferred among the various carriers (18).

In the absence of an exogenous carrier, several streptococcal chains which possess CBH may possibly attach themselves to the surface of a cell. Upon transfer of the hemolytic moiety, the cell membrane undergoes permeability changes which eventually lead to cell death (21).

Both SLO and SLS activities are strongly inhibited by lipids (16, 18, 22, 23). While SLO is a strong immunogen and induces the formation of precipitating and neutralizing antibodies (16), SLS is apparently non-immunogenic (18, 23).

Mammalian cells affected by either SLO or SLS undergo rapid swelling and lysis. The cells lose many of their macromolecular components and die (21, 23, 24). Cell damage is thought to be induced by the interaction of the hemolysins with some phospholipid structure of the cell membrane. Thus, SLO may "punch holes" in the membranes (16, 18, 23), whereas SLS probably disorients some lipid structures of the membranes without actually making "holes" (18). An alternative suggestion is that both SLO and SLS rupture the cell membrane of the lysosome (23–25), and that the release of hydrolytic enzymes from the granules brings about lysis of intracellular organelles and subsequent death of the cells. The majority of the lysosomal enzymes have pH optima of 4.5 to 5.5, which probably is the range of pH developing in foci of streptococcal proliferation. Thus, "activation" of lysosomal enzymes by lactic acid produced by the streptococcus may contribute greatly to the damaging effect of streptococcal metabolites on the host tissues (24–26). Since they kill leukocytes, both SLO and SLS may be classified as "virulence factors" and together with the M-protein and hyaluronic acid may greatly contribute to the invasiveness and long persistence of streptococci in tissues (1, 27).

Large amounts of SLO and SLS, released in the immediate vicinity of streptococci, may contribute not only to local tissue damage, but may ultimately reach target cells remote from their site of release, when they diffuse into the blood and lymph.

Most of our knowledge of the tissue-damaging properties of these two hemolysins comes from experiments with laboratory animals.

The i.v. injection of SLS leads to massive intravascular hemolysis and acute necrosis of the liver in mice and rabbits (28, 29). I.p. injection of SLS into mice results in tubular necrosis of the kidney (30); and intra-articular injection of SLS in rabbits causes severe arthritis (31, 32). I.v. injections of SLO cause only very slight hemolysis in mice but a proportion of the animals die within a few minutes (16, 23, 33).

One of the most prominent characteristics of SLO is its distinct cardio-

toxicity. The toxin can effect the contraction of the heart and cause
constriction of the coronary arteries, and can also induce cerebral damage
(16, 23, 34, 35). SLO may cause tissue damage through the formation
of immune complexes, which may be deposited in tissues and initiate
immune-complex injury (16). SLO may also injure the heart muscle by
sensitizing it to an anaphylactic reaction if adequate amounts of circulating anti-SLO antibodies are present (36).

Although none of the pathological alterations induced in animals by
streptococcal hemolysins resembles those seen in human beings with poststreptococcal complications, both hemolytic substances may participate
in more complicated mechanisms of tissue damage, which may in turn
lead to the development of poststreptococcal diseases (see below).

2) *Spreading factors: proteinase, streptokinase, hyaluronidase and the
nucleases.* Streptococci usually cause infections which tend to spread
through the tissues, inducing cellulitis. Streptococcal spread usually involves the dissolution and depolymerization of the ground substance of
connective tissue, as well as lysis of the protein and the nucleic acid
matrix which forms following the clotting of blood or the accumulation
of lysed tissue cells at the site of inflammation.

Most group A streptococci elaborate a proteolytic enzyme which is
secreted as a precursor and is activated when the pH of the milieu drops
below 6.8, or when abundant reducing substances (SH-groups) or traces
of proteolytic enzymes are available (37–39). This proteinase, which has
many properties similar to papain, can digest numerous proteins and
peptides, including the streptococcus' own protein antigens (40) (see
below). The enzyme also acts upon mucopolysaccharides of connective
tissue, to split chondroitin sulfate and hyaluronic acid (41). The i.v.
injection of the proteinase into rabbits, mice and guinea pigs induces
severe myocardial and skeletal-muscle necrosis (42). The extensive lesions
are sometimes calcified and, in the case of the heart, are not confined
to any particular region. The severity of the lesions is greatest in the heart,
and in other muscles appears to parallel the extent of normal mechanical
activity. The proteinase acts synergistically with SLS to destroy mammalian
cells (43). Whereas it cannot injure intact cells, it readily penetrates injured ones, causing intracellular digestion. It may thus exacerbate tissue
damage by the further activation and release of lysosomal enzymes (43).
It is thus apparent that the release and activation of proteinase in and
around foci of streptococcal proliferation *in vivo* may greatly contribute
to tissue injury and to the invasiveness of the bacteria.

Most group A streptococci elaborate another factor which may aid the spread of infection in the tissues in a similar manner. Streptococcal cultures have long been known to lyse blood clots. This property was at first thought to be due to the release of a fibrinolytic enzyme by the streptococcus, splitting both fibrinogen and fibrin (44). The organism was later shown to synthesize an extracellular factor, termed streptokinase (SK) which, by itself, is not proteolytic (45). In interacts, however, with a proenzyme, plasminogen, found in human serum, and converts it to a proteolytic enzyme, plasmin, which digests fibrinogen, fibrin and a variety of other proteins in the blood and connective tissue (46).

The presence of proteolytic enzymes in close proximity to streptococci *in vivo* may prevent the host from walling off the bacteria by plasma clots formed in the process of inflammation. The enzymes may also act upon the connective tissue matrix, deplete protein in cartilage and mucopolysaccharides (47) and cause increased vascular permeability (48). It is of interest that SK preparations are extensively used by clinicians to help lyse intravascular clots and for the débridement of necrotic wounds.

The relationship between SK production and streptococcal virulence has been much debated. Since SK is also produced by streptococci of Groups C and G, which are only slightly virulent in man, its function as a virulence factor is dubious. Studies on the possible contribution of the SK-plasmin system to the virulence of streptococci in laboratory animal models have been hampered by the fact that the blood of many animals lacks some of the components of the fibrinolytic system of human beings. Thus, the addition of human plasminogen is required for the activation by SK of the proteolytic system in rabbit serum. Microorganisms which do not usually produce SK can better invade host tissues if they are suspended in SK-plasminogen mixtures (49–51).

Plasmin can exert adverse effects on the animal organism very similar to the effects of streptococcal proteinases, causing cardiac and muscular lesions (52). It can also inactivate serum complement, which enhances the phagocytosis of a variety of microorganisms (53).

Spread of streptococci in the tissue may also be enhanced by the destruction of hyaluronic acid of the connective tissue by the extracellular enzyme hyaluronidase, produced by many group A strains (54). Hyaluronidase depolymerizes hyaluronic acid by splitting glucose amidic bonds to yield oligosaccharides. Production of hyaluronidase by the streptococcus also results in the destruction of the hyaluronic capsule around the streptococci. This factor is probably identical with the "spreading factor" described by Duran-Reynals (55) and is believed by many workers to enhance not only the spread of streptococcal infections in tissues, but also of infections caused by a variety of other microorganisms (56). However, some investigators have found no parallelism between hyaluronidase production *in vitro* and the dissemination of streptococci in the animal. On the other hand, strains producing large amounts of the enzyme are more lethal to chick embryos than strains producing none (57). Protection of mice against infection with streptococci has been effected by repeated injections of leech extracts containing hyaluronidase, suggesting that the hyaluronic acid capsule plays a role in the virulence of the organisms.

The spread of streptococci in tissues may also be enhanced by the secretion of deoxyribonuclease (DNase) and ribonuclease (RNase), which lyse the thick, purulent exudate accumulating at the site of inflammation in the tissues (58, 59). This exudate is usually composed of a viscous DNA-RNA matrix derived from injured tissue cells. At least four antigenic varieties of DNase have been described (60). This enzyme is produced by all streptococcal types tested, and DNase degradation products are believed to serve as nutritional supplements for virulent streptococci (61), in addition to facilitating their spread.

3) *The antimetabolic factor NAD-glycohydrolase.* Many group A streptococcal strains produce NAD-glycohydrolase (NADase) (62), which can destroy NAD and may thus affect the oxidative metabolism of the host cells (63). The possible role played by this enzyme in the destruction of leukocytes has been extensively studied. Almost all streptococcal strains which synthesize NADase are capable of killing leukocytes following phagocytosis ("leukotoxicity") (64, 65). In contrast, strains not producing NADase consistently fail to exert leukotoxic effects. It was therefore thought that leukotoxicity involves the intracellular release of NADase by the engulfed streptococcus, leading to paralysis of the metabolic apparatus of the leukocyte. Thus, this enzyme may be classified as one of the virulence factors of streptococci.

More recently, it has been postulated that the leukotoxic factor is instead associated with CBH (SLS in its cell-bound form) (66), on the basis of the following observations: Leukotoxicity and SLS production are both associated with young cultures in the logarithmic growth phase. Such young cultures were screened for NADase and SLS production. It was found, surprisingly, that all strains not producing NADase, which were nonleukotoxic, consistently failed to synthesize SLS in the early logarithmic phase of growth. If, on the other hand, the same strains were harvested from the stationary phase of growth, they produced large amounts of SLS and were leukotoxic. Moreover, a streptococcus mutant which produced large amounts of NADase, but failed to synthesize SLS in any phase of growth, was not leukotoxic. Thus, the leukotoxic factor produced by group A streptococci is probably identical with SLS. All the NADase-free strains fail to synthesize a cell-bound lipoproteinase (67), and these strains may also prove to differ from the regular strains in other biological properties. The possibility that NADase itself may contribute to the intracellular killing of leukocytes is not, however, ruled out.

4) *Erythrogenic toxins.* Many streptococcal strains elaborate a group of extracellular erythrogenic toxins which exert a distinct toxic effect on a variety of mammalian tissues, and modify the host responses to a variety of injurious agents.

Some patients with upper respiratory infections due to group A streptococci develop scarlet fever. This disease is characterized by the appearance of multiple rashes which usually appear several days following the onset of infection. Streptococcal strains isolated from such patients produce a toxin, or toxins, known as the erythrogenic toxin (68). For years, this toxin was thought to exert its effects on blood vessel endothelium, causing diapedesis of red blood cells and thereby the characteristic rash. This effect of the toxin can be neutralized by convalescent serum, or by the serum of animals immunized with the toxin. Injection of antitoxin into the rash area results in a blanching effect known as the Schultz-Carlton effect (1, 68). Since the injection of the toxin into normal animals seldom causes any rash, and since children under the age of six seldom develop scarlet fever, it was postulated that the skin rash of scarlet fever may be linked to a hypersensitivity state which develops only as a result of repeated exposure to streptococci.

For many years, interest in scarlet fever toxins was very limited. Renewed attention has recently been focused on the toxins by the observation that they are formed in large amounts only after the streptococcus has interacted with its host *in vivo*, and that they have many other biological properties in addition to the ability to induce rashes (69, 70).

When streptococci are injected into the skin of rabbits, they induce edematous skin lesions which readily spread through the dermis (cellulitis) (71). An extract of the skin lesions enhances the lethal and cardiotoxic properties of SLO (71) and of gram-negative bacterial endotoxins

(70). Injections of such a skin lesion extract 3 hr prior to the injection of erythrogenic toxin also markedly enhances its lethality. I.c. injection of streptococci into rabbits modifies the animals' subsequent response to streptococci given intranasally, which then persists in the lungs, myocardium and the lymphatic system for many months (69). The factor present in the skin lesions was identified as erythrogenic toxin (69).

Purified erythrogenic toxin is cytotoxic to macrophages (69, 70), and toxins produced *in vivo* prepare the animals for a Shwartzman phenomenon evoked by bacterial endotoxins or by SLO (71).

Erythrogenic toxin is pyrogenic (72). Small amounts cause a very steep rise in fever, which can be inhibited by cortisone. Another property of the toxin is its skin reactivity, manifested by a delayed hypersensitivity reaction in animals previously exposed to streptococci or to the purified toxin. This reactivity can be passively transferred to another animal by lymphocytes (73). These observations underline the probability that the skin rash seen in scarlet fever patients is the result of the development of a delayed hypersensitivity reaction. Finally, the erythrogenic toxin is capable of blocking the function of the RES (64) and of suppressing the primary immune response of animals to certain antigens (69, 74).

Despite the many biological activities demonstrated for the erythrogenic toxin in laboratory animals, very little is as yet known about its role in the pathogenesis of streptococcal diseases in human beings.

5) *Cardiohepatic toxins.* When living streptococci of high virulence are injected into susceptible animals, septicemia terminating fatally within a few days usually ensues. The lesions are widespread, affect most of the parenchymatous organs and resemble those described in patients who die of scarlet fever after having survived more than 10 days following infection. When streptococci of low virulence are injected into the tonsils of rabbits, the animals develop acute myocardial lesions within 72 hr (75, 76). In these lesions, necrotic foci are infiltrated with mononuclear cells, and some of the lesions later develop into giant-cell granulomas. Since similar, but more severe, lesions can be induced in rabbits by the intratonsillar injection of a concentrated supernate derived from streptococcal cultures, it is assumed that extracellular streptococcal products may also be responsible for the initiation of tissue damage following the intratonsillar administration of the bacteria (76, 77). The extracellular products also cause severe granulomatous lesions of the diaphragm and the liver, in addition to the heart lesions.

The nature of the "toxin" present in the culture supernate is not known, but its low mol wt differentiates it from many of the streptococcal exotoxins (78). Like other streptococcal toxins, this low molecular weight agent may prepare tissues for the localization of streptococci (see Section D 2).

6) *Nephrotoxins.* A few of the 60 group A streptococcal types known today have been associated with outbreaks of acute glomerulonephritis (AGN) in human beings (12, 79). This association was recently established by epidemiological and clinical studies (80), but little is known about the mechanisms by which such nephritogenic types initiate AGN.

The fact that only a limited number of group A strains (types 12, 49, 55, 57) are associated with AGN points to the elaboration by such strains of a specific nephrotoxin responsible for renal damage. On the other hand, the similarity between streptococcal glomerulonephritis in man and the "immune complex" nephritis induced in experimental animals following immunization with foreign proteins (81, 82) suggests that AGN following streptococcal infections may also be caused by the deposition in the kidneys of immune complexes consisting of certain streptococcal antigens and host antibodies.

Kidney lesions can commonly be induced in a variety of laboratory animals by the repeated inoculation of nephritogenic streptococci, or by their implantation in diffusion chambers in the peritoneal cavity (83, 84). Tubular necrosis with very mild glomerular alterations accompanied by hematuria and albuminuria ensue. In some cases, however, the tubular lesions have been attributed to SLS which is elaborated by both nephritogenic and non-nephritogenic streptococci (30).

Rabbits inoculated s.c. with type 12 streptococci isolated from a nephritic patient develop severe hypertension and moderate hematuria 17 days later. Similar results are obtained after treatment with culture filtrates of these microorganisms (85, 86). Non-nephritogenic streptococci fail to induce such lesions. The affected animals develop tubular lesions of the type associated with lower nephron nephritis, and mild glomerular lesions which consist of dilatation and congestion of capillaries. On the other hand, in rhesus monkeys receiving crude nephrotoxin derived from dialysates of type 12 streptococcal cultures, the capsular epithelium of the glomeruli proliferates and the capillary basement membrane thickens (87). The lesions progress from the acute to the subacute phase, and epithelial crescents similar to those seen in human beings with AGN are prevalent. Thus, different animal species react differently to the nephrotoxin.

The nephrotoxic substance in the culture supernates of nephritogenic streptococci is claimed to be a low mol wt peptide (88) with no direct effect on tissue cultures of kidney cells (89). Its mode of action *in vivo* is not known.

Other workers have shown that both an "autolysate" (90) and sonicates (91) of washed type 12 streptococci induce severe hypertension, proteinuria and pathological alterations in the glomeruli of rabbits. The nature of these nephrotoxins is not known, but they probably differ from the low mol wt toxin found in culture supernates. The mode of action of these nephrotoxins is also unknown, but they are thought to exert a direct damaging effect on the kidney, which may later trigger more complicated immunopathological episodes leading to chronic renal damage.

7) *Antiphagocytic agents: M-protein and hyaluronic acid.* One of the most important determinants of the relations between the streptococcus and its host is the integrity and efficiency of the latter's RES.

Leukocytes are known not to approach certain virulent streptococci. In other instances, however, an encounter between the two types of cell results in prompt phagocytosis of the streptococci. If sera of patients convalescing from an infection with the same streptococcal strain are preincubated with the streptococci, the microorganisms are rapidly phagocytosed. Something in the patient's serum appears to abolish the antiphagocytic properties of the streptococcus. If streptococci with antiphagocytic properties are pretreated with trypsin, they also rapidly lose their antiphagocytic attributes. The antiphagocytic property of the streptococcus is associated with the type-specific surface antigen, the M-protein, considered to be one of the main virulence factors of these bacteria (9).

The M-protein has a multimolecular structure (92), is soluble in alcohol and resistant to boiling at pH 2.0 (9), but is readily inactivated by many proteolytic enzymes, including the streptococcus' own proteolytic systems (9). The efficient elimination of streptococci from the tissues depends largely on the synthesis of type-specific anti-M antibodies, which neutralize its antiphagocytic powers. Thus, any vaccine against streptococci must include the purified M-proteins of the most common types of streptococcus prevalent in a community (93). The acquisition of type-specific immunity also depends largely on whether or not the patients had received early treatment with antibiotics. Thus, the early elimination of streptococci from the upper respiratory tract diminishes the chances of developing adequate titers of anti-M antibodies, and reinfection with the same type of streptococcus is therefore likely to occur. On the other hand, delay of antibiotic therapy carries with it the obvious danger that some of the patients may develop rheumatic fever or nephritis.

The precise mechanisms by which antibodies to the M-protein contribute to the destruction of the streptococcus are still not clear. Gram-positive microorganisms are not usually susceptible to immune lysis. It is more likely that by combining with the M-protein on the surface of the streptococcus, the antibodies change their surface charge, and thereby permit attraction of phagocytes and subsequent phagocytosis.

Many streptococcal strains synthesize a nonimmunogenic, superficial, capsular polysaccharide (hyaluronic acid), a copolymer of NAGA and D-glucuronic acid (4, 94). The capsule confers a mucoid appearance on the streptococcus. As the bacteria age, the capsular material disappears from their surface and may be found in the culture medium. The disappearance of the capsule is usually associated with the synthesis of hyaluronidase by the streptococcus (54).

The role played by the hyaluronic acid capsule in streptococcal infections is still not fully understood, but it is assumed that the virulence of group A streptococci for laboratory animals is due in part to its presence (95, 96). Hyaluronic acid may well be the main virulence factor of group C streptococci, which do not produce M-protein. It is believed by some workers that hyaluronic acid may aid in establishing the streptococcus in the nasopharynx, while the M-protein determines the later course of infection (97). Hyaluronic acid may contribute to the invasiveness of streptococci by impeding phagocytosis, and, like M-protein, can thus be considered to be a "virulence factor" (98). Capsular hyaluronic acid also interferes with the attachment of bacteriophage to the streptococcal cells (99).

By the selective action of some virulent phages on cultures of susceptible streptococci, it is possible to alter or enhance certain of the streptococcal characteristics. Thus, nonmucoid strains become mucoid, with or without an increase in M-protein. Certain nonlysogenic streptococci, which failed to produce erythrogenic toxin, also acquire this ability when they are infected by a temperature phage isolated from known scarlatinal toxin-producing strains (100). Production of this toxin is apparently related to the synthesis of mature phage particles, since ultraviolet enhancement of phage production results in a concomitant increase in toxin titer. Whether a similar phage-bacterium relationship exists *in vivo* remains to be determined.

D) CELLULAR INJURY DUE TO DEGRADATION OF THE STREPTOCOCCUS
IN THE TISSUES

1) *The role of phagocytosis.* The fate of the streptococcus following its phagocytosis determines its survival in the host and the realization of its pathogenic potential.

Very shortly after phagocytosis by granulocytes, streptococci are found within membrane-lined phagocytic vacuoles known as phagosomes. Fusion between the phagosome and the lysosomes results in the secretion by the latter of numerous hydrolytic enzymes with a pH optimum of approximately 5.0, which presumably are able to attack cell wall components of the bacteria (101).

Little is known of the enzymatic steps leading to degradation of group A streptococci. Electron micrographs taken several hours following phagocytosis show that, although the morphology of the majority of the cocci is altered beyond recognition, several organisms always remain intact within the phagosomes (102). No enzymatic system capable of completely degrading the streptococcal cell wall components *in vitro* has yet been isolated from phagocytic cells (103, 104). Since injection of intact streptococci into animal tissues usually results in the initiation of a prolonged inflammatory process, accompanied by the persistence of cell-wall components in the inflammatory areas, it is assumed that mammalian tissues probably do not contain efficient muralytic systems capable of rapidly and completely degrading the cell walls of group A streptococci.

The recent demonstration of the enzyme N-acetylglucosaminidase in macrophages of rabbits and human beings (104) may explain how the serological specificity of streptococcal polysaccharide antigens changes from the A-specificity (directed against the terminal NAGA of the C-polysaccharide) to that of the A-variant (directed against the rhamnosyl-mucopeptide) remaining after the removal of the terminal N-acetylglucosamide. Thus, human beings infected with streptococci develop antibodies to the A-specificity in the early phase of immunization, and against A-variant specificity at a later stage (105). However, removal of NAGA from the C-polysaccharide by the N-acetylglucosaminidase without the removal of the rhamnose residues does not permit the cleavage of the remaining mucopeptide by tissue lysozyme (106). As the majority of streptococci are ultimately degraded within the leukocytes, it seems probable that certain leukocytes do possess muralytic enzymes capable of breaking the rigid skeleton of the streptococcus, although such enzymes would appear to be of low efficiency.

2) *Persistence of streptococcal products in the initiation of chronic inflammation.* When streptococcal cell wall fragments are injected into the skin of rabbits, they incite an inflammatory process which may persist for many months (106–110). The lesions are granulomatous and tend to relapse, so that secondary and tertiary nodular lesions appear and disappear at the site of the primary lesion. The pathological process affects the connective tissue and intercellular ground substance, and is characterized by the infiltration of numerous mononuclear phagocytes. The toxic bacterial elements responsible are associated with the macromolecular complex of polysaccharide and protein. The group-specific C-polysaccharide is an essential part of the toxic complex.

As long as the inflammatory process continues, fluorescent antibodies to the streptococcal cell walls demonstrate cell wall remnants within phagocytes at the inflammatory sites (106, 107). Once the inflammatory process is resolved, no traces of streptococcal antigen can be demonstrated in the area. Thus, persistence of the antigen is related to continuation of the inflammation. On the other hand, if the streptococcal cell wall is degraded *in vitro* by muralytic enzymes derived from *Streptomyces albus* or from the phage lysates of group C streptococci (107), the cell wall fragments disappear very quickly from the tissues without causing chronic inflammation. Moreover, no chronic and relapsing nodules are induced by bacterial species readily lysed by macrophage enzymes.

When streptococcal cell fragments containing C-polysaccharide-mucopeptide complexes are injected into the knee joints of rabbits, the animals develop severe arthritis, and cell-wall fragments can be detected for many weeks at the site of the lesions (109). Mice inoculated i.v. with streptococcal cell-wall fragments develop heart lesions said to be similar to those in rheumatic fever patients (100, 111).

Cell-wall remnants are demonstrable with the aid of fluorescent antibodies within phagocytic cells in the heart lesions. Although the route by which these fragments reach the heart is not known, recent observations may shed light on this process. A single injection of washed streptococci into the myocardium of rabbits results in the development of giant-cell granulomas which bear some resemblance to the lesions found in human beings following streptococcal infections (112). Neither damage of the heart muscle in the absence of streptococci, nor the injection of streptococci i.v. results in the formation of such lesions. On the other hand, when the i.v. injection of streptococci is preceded by physical trauma to the heart, granulomatous lesions develop at the site of the injury, in-

dicating that tissue damage predisposes to the localization of streptococci. This suggests that if circulating streptococcal toxins injure the
heart, streptococci may subsequently localize at the site of the toxin
injury.

Indeed, rabbits first injected with the cardiohepatic toxins and then
challenged i.p. or intratonsillarly with fluorescein-labeled streptococci, develop cardiac lesions which contain many macrophages loaded with
labeled bacteria (113). Similarly, labeled streptococci localize in the liver
(113) and joints (114) of rabbits previously injured by SLS or by
bacterial sonicates. Moreover, the microorganisms also migrate within
phagocytic cells to tissue sites previously damaged by delayed hypersensitivity reactions (113). To explain how the streptococci reach the
damaged sites, it was postulated that tissue injury generates chemotactic
factors which attract phagocytic cells. Macrophages which have engulfed
streptococci either in the tonsils or in the peritoneum may thus translocate them to the damaged tissues. Upon arrival at the lesions, the degradation products of the streptococcal cell walls may incite a secondary
inflammation. Cell wall fragments persisting in tissue in intact or partially degraded form would then contribute to the perpetuation of the
chronic inflammatory reaction. However, it remains to be proved experimentally that the arrival of cocci-laden macrophages to tissue sites
previously damaged by toxin can indeed trigger such a sequence of
events.

The long persistence of streptococcal products in the tissues raises the
possibility that different phagocytes may possess different types of lysosomal enzyme participating in the intracellular degradation of the bacteria
(27, 101). Thus, the fate of the streptococcus following phagocytosis
would depend considerably on the type of leukocyte first encountered.
Rheumatic fever patients may perhaps lack one or more of the key
enzymes which degrade the streptococcal cell walls to non-noxious entities
(27), and the disease may thus perhaps derive from an error of host
metabolism.

Another streptococcal cell wall component is a mucopeptide, very toxic
to a variety of mammalian cell systems (7). This mucopeptide, which
constitutes the rigid skeleton of the organism, can cause marked inflammatory reactions in the skin of animals. When injected i.v., it causes
severe granulomatous lesions in the heart. Prominent among its biological properties are its pyrogenicity and its capacity to prepare animals
for the Shwartzman phenomenon. Like endotoxins of gram-negative

microorganisms, the streptococcal mucopeptide enhances the resistance of mice to subsequent challenge with virulent streptococci. It can also inhibit phagocytosis of bacteria by polymorphonuclear leukocytes, and is cytotoxic to tissue culture cells. Thus, the release of mucopeptide from the streptococcal cells following their degradation by macrophages may greatly enhance the toxicity of the streptococcus to a variety of tissues.

E) INJURY TO THE HOST INITIATED BY THE IMMUNE RESPONSE TO STREPTOCOCCI

Tissue injury in streptococcal infections of man may be initiated by a variety of immunological mechanisms, in addition to the directly toxic action of the bacterium. Thus, cardiac and arthritic lesions, similar to those seen in rheumatic fever patients, and renal lesions, similar to those of AGN, develop in laboratory animals after repeated exposure to foreign proteins (115). Tissue damage in the organism may therefore result from hypersensitivity reactions, of both the immediate and the delayed type, and immunological cross-reactivity between streptococcal and tissue antigens may carry a share of the responsibility.

1) *The role of passive immune sensitization.* Allogeneic and heterogeneic mammalian cells are lysed by immune serum in the presence of complement. This is direct immune lysis. Indirect immune lysis may also take place through the agency of antibodies directed at antigens coating the cell surface, and streptococcal antigens can sensitize tissue cells to such indirect destruction.

Many streptococcal strains produce a cell-sensitizing factor (SF) (116–119) which has a strong affinity for the membranes of a variety of mammalian cells. Cells sensitized with this antigen are destroyed in the presence of convalescent serum containing a high titer of antibodies against the SF (116). SF introduced into the joints of normal animals elicits no pathological alterations (120). On the other hand, when SF is injected intra-articularly into rabbits previously immunized with killed streptococci, severe arthritis occurs (120).

The SF is a hapten and is immunogenic when coupled to certain carriers found naturally on streptococcal cells. The capacity of such haptens to cause pathological immune reactions is probably similar to that of certain haptenic drugs which, when coupled to cell membrane components, can cause severe hemolytic anemias and other lesions.

2) *The role of cross-reactive antigens.* An antigenic similarity between

certain streptococcal substances and components of heart, kidney, and connective tissue of man has long been recognized. When a human being is exposed to streptococci, some of the antibodies which the host develops against the invader may therefore also interact with the cross-reactive antigens of his own tissues and severe tissue damage may ensue (121, 122). At least two groups of streptococcal antigens cross-reactive with heart (121, 122), and one each with kidney (123) and connective tissue (124) have been observed.

Streptococcal antigens cross-reactive with heart are found both in the bacterial cell wall and cell membrane (121, 122). Whereas the cell wall-associated cross-reactive antigen has been detected in only six Group A types, antigen localized in the bacterial membrane is common to all Group A types tested (121). Immunization of rabbits with intact strep-tococci and cell membranes of Groups A and C shows that whereas almost all Group A strains share a common antigen with the heart, only a few of the Group C streptococci possess such an antigen.

The kidney-related streptococcal antigens are associated with the bacterial cell membrane (123) and the microbial antigens cross-reactive with connective tissue are related to the group-specific polysaccharide of the cell wall (121, 124).

If rheumatic fever and nephritis really are caused by the interaction of cross-reactive antibodies with tissue components, such antibodies should localize in the affected tissues. Although γ-globulins and com-plement were found to be concentrated in the sarcolemma and subsarco-lemma of cardiac myofibers in five children who died of acute rheumatic fever (122), very little deposition of immunoglobulins was evident in the Aschoff bodies characteristic of the rheumatic lesion in the heart. The widespread deposition of immunoglobulin and complement was thought to be related to the cardiac failure and abnormal electrocardiographic changes recorded in these patients. It is not known whether the im-munoglobulins localized in the heart were induced by streptococcal antigens cross-reactive with cardiac components, and no data are as yet available on the cytotoxicity of such cross-reactive antibodies to heart muscle *in vitro* or *in vivo*. It remains an open question whether the observed cardiac lesions are triggered by such antibodies, or whether the antibodies are made only after injury to the heart by other agents, for example strep-tococcal toxins. Although higher titers of cross-reactive antiheart anti-bodies have been found consistently in rheumatic fever patients as com-pared with patients recovering without sequelae from acute streptococcal infections (125), the presence of such antibodies in the latter group raises some doubts as to their pathogenic role.

A common glycoprotein antigen has been isolated from nephritic kidneys and streptococcal membranes (126). Immunization of rabbits with an extract prepared from the membranes of nephritogenic streptococci leads to the development of nephrotoxic antibodies which cause glomerular lesions and proteinuria in rats (127). It remains to be demonstrated whether the serum of nephritic patients is cytotoxic to normal human kidney cells.

While cross-reactive immunity may be responsible at least in part for the pathogenesis of chronic streptococcal disease of man, it would be premature to view this theory as the sole or major explanation.

3) *The role of immune complexes.* Another likely mechanism of tissue damage involving immunological reactions is the formation and deposition in tissue of immune complexes between certain streptococcal antigens and their antibodies.

Immune complexes are known to trigger severe inflammatory reactions of the Arthus type (81, 128, 129) and complexes formed in antigen excess are especially irritating. Such complexes may cause the release of pharmacological agents from certain tissue cells, may fix complement and may lead to the generation of chemotactic factors. The mechanisms of their formation have been studied, mainly in relation to the induction of nephritis, carditis and arthritis following the development of serum sickness in animals immunized with foreign proteins (115, 128, 129). Animals with high titers of circulating antibodies to foreign protein do not generally develop immunopathological complications, whereas poor antibody producers frequently show severe tissue lesions. The trapping of such complexes in tissues such as heart, joints and kidneys undoubtedly directly results in the induction of acute local inflammation. The antigen concentrated in the complexes may also be directly injurious, apart from the damage caused by the complexes themselves. In addition, polymorphonuclear leukocytes (PMN) rich in lysosomes are attracted to such tissue sites. Phagocytosis of the immune complexes by the PMN is accompanied by release into the tissues of hydrolytic enzymes from the lysosome, which may initiate still further tissue damage (130).

Antibodies to streptococcal M-protein can be eluted from the glomeruli of rats carrying i.p. diffusion chambers containing nephritogenic streptococci (131, 132). M-protein is also localized in the kidneys of human beings who have developed poststreptococcal nephritis (133). The route by which the M-protein reaches the kidney is unknown. The protein may possibly be stripped off the streptococcus by macrophages (134) either in the tonsils or in the skin, and may be transported to the kidney, already complexed with immune globulins. On the other hand, streptococci causing nephritis may localize in the glomeruli due to preceding injury by a nephrotoxin (88, 90, 91). M-protein might then be removed *in situ* where it could combine with antibodies. To complicate matters, M-protein can also form complexes with fibrinogen, and such complexes may also be trapped by the kidney and cause renal damage (135, 136). More recently, it has been postulated that AGN may be caused by the deposition in the kidney of plasma membrane constituents of certain nephritogenic streptococci (137). Such membrane components can form complexes with antimembrane antibodies, with fixation of complement and subsequent immune complex injury.

Immune complexes of streptococcal products have also been suspected of initiating heart lesions. Rabbits immunized with C-polysaccharide develop no pathological lesions. On the other hand, polysaccharide coupled with the protein edestin induces the formation of precipitating antibodies, and the immunized animals develop severe necrotic lesions of the myocardium and heart valves (138). The suspicion that similar immune complexes in human beings may possibly precipitate in the heart muscle to cause tissue damage should be studied. The C-polysaccharides of group A streptococci share common antigens with mucopolysaccharide of the connective tissue of various mammals (124, 138), and this cross-reactive immunity may thus play a role in the pathogenesis of connective tissue damage.

F) ROLE OF STREPTOCOCCAL L-FORMS

Streptococci can exist in the animal body as entities devoid of a cell wall, the L-forms (139). There may be considerable survival value in the organism's ability to modulate its form in this direction. Thus, it is known that bacteria treated with penicillin may convert into protoplasts or L-forms. These structures, surrounded by a phospholipid membrane, lack most of the components of the cell wall, but can multiply readily both *in vitro* and *in vivo* and can continue to synthesize many of the antigens expressed by the intact organisms (140). One of the advantages which the L-form has over the parent strain is its nonsensitivity to penicillin, the antibiotic of choice for the treatment of streptococcal infection.

Since some of the L-forms may spontaneously revert to the parent strain, their persistence in tissues may constitute a source for "reinfection" of the same individual. L-forms can exist over many cell generations within the cytoplasm of certain mammalian cells in tissue culture (141), and *in vivo* in mice (142), without damaging the cells. Their intracellular location protects them against the deleterious effects of antibodies.

The causes and mechanisms of the reversible conversions between the parent strain and L-forms are still not understood, nor is it known whether L-forms as such are pathogenic for human beings. It has been claimed that monkeys receiving repeated intratonsillar inoculations of streptococcal L-forms develop carditis and encephalitis (143), and that the cardiac damage following such inoculation of L-forms is similar to that seen after intratonsillar injection of viable intact streptococci (75–78). The L-forms may thus release toxic substances which diffuse and reach the heart and brain. Alternatively, since L-forms may possess membrane antigens cross-reactive with heart (121), cardiac damage may be caused by cross-reactive cytotoxic antibodies (122). Since patients with streptococcal infections are treated with large doses of penicillin, it is theoretically possible that L-forms may be involved in the persistence of streptococci in the host, and may thus contribute to the pathogenesis of poststreptococcal sequelae.

G) CONCLUDING REMARKS AND SUMMARY

Some of the biological mechanisms by which streptococci persist in the tissues and cause damage in the host have been described. Much of the available information comes from animal models and although it is likely that similar mechanisms are responsible for the pathology of streptococcal infection in man, much further work is necessary to substantiate this view.

There appear to exist two distinct modes of immediate and long-range streptococcal pathogenicity. First, a variety of streptococcal products can initiate direct toxic effects on the tissues of the host. The persistence and slow degradation of the streptococcus in the tissues is assumed to be the major cause for the chronic pathologic sequelae of acute infection. Second, a variety of immune reactions may initiate the disease processes. These mechanisms are not mutually exclusive and a combination of both may best explain streptococcal disease syndromes (14, 27, 144).

The events which take place in the tissues of nonimmunized animals exposed to group A streptococci are undoubtedly different from those occurring in animals presensitized to the pathogen.

In nonimmunized animals, the invading streptococcus probably at first encounters only low host resistance. The rapid proliferation of the microorganisms in the tonsils or elsewhere can be expected to lead to the formation of large amounts of a variety of toxic agents. When leukocytes approach such a focus of streptococcal proliferation, they have to traverse a milieu containing gradients of increasing toxin concentration. Thus, crippling of the phagocytic system by leukocidins at the site of entry of the streptococcus may be of crucial significance for the outcome of the infection. M-protein and hyaluronic acid upon the surface of the bacterium also impede phagocytosis, and enhance bacterial multiplication and, thereby, toxin production. Spread of streptococci can be considerably facilitated by the conversion of plasminogen to plasmin by SK, and by the secretion of hyaluronidase and proteinase, which help to degrade the connective tissue matrix and lead to further tissue destruction. The production of streptococcal hemolysins capable of disrupting lysosomes may also contribute to the initiation of tissue damage *in situ*.

Streptococcal toxins eventually spread through the bloodstream and lymphatics, and can cause severe damage to cells at sites remote from the portal of entry of the pathogen. SLO can affect cardiac function and can lead to myocarditis. SLS and the nephrotoxins may, upon reaching the kidney, cause tubular necrosis and glomerular injury, and erythrogenic toxin, cardiohepatic toxin and proteinase can lead to myocardial and hepatic necrosis.

By elaborating erythrogenic toxins, the streptococcus can modify the host response to further challenge with either SLO or with bacterial endotoxins, causing Shwartzman reactions and also enhancing the persistence of streptococci in tissues. Both the erythrogenic toxin and fractions containing mucopeptide may elicit pyrogenic effects. These agents may also directly damage the heart muscle and may weaken the host response by exerting toxic effects on the RES, suppressing phagocytosis and perhaps delaying the development of an immune response to the streptococcus.

Streptococci are eventually phagocytosed, especially after they have lost their M-protein due to proteolysis at the site of inflammation. Macrophages and granulocytes which have engulfed the organisms may then destroy them directly or translocate them either to the RES centers where they are disposed of, or to remote tissue sites (i.e., heart, liver, joints, etc.) which may have been injured by streptococcal toxins or other agents. Eventual degradation of the streptococcal cell walls at these sites releases toxic cell-wall moieties which may elicit and perpetuate a chronic inflammatory response. Persistence of streptococcal components in the tissues and perpetuation of inflammation depend on whether leukocyte enzymes can eventually degrade the cell-wall components to non-noxious fragments.

The host may either succumb to the acute infection with streptococcal septicemia, or survive. Some of the survivors develop chronic sequelae which may affect a variety of vital organs. If the surviving individual is again attacked by the same streptococcal strain, he is likely to respond fairly rapidly, at least to some of the streptococcal antigens, with a secondary immune response. The antibodies are able to neutralize SLO and other cytotoxic antigens which interfere with phagocytosis. Antibodies against M-protein, the major virulence factor, enhance phagocytosis and elimination of the microorganisms from the tissues, and the infection often remains limited and mild. By way of contrast, secondary infection with a streptococcal type different from that first encountered is often characterized by rapid proliferation of the microorganisms, owing to the absence of type-specific immunity. Although there may be antibodies to some antigenically similar streptococcal exoproducts, these alone may be incapable of offering categorical protection against reinfection.

Streptococcal antigens probably form complexes with antibodies in the circulation. In poor antibody producers, the immune complexes tend to be of the soluble type in the zone of antigen excess, and may initiate extensive damage to connective tissues and kidneys, similar to that in animals sensitized to foreign proteins. The development of cellular hypersensitivity to a variety of streptococcal antigens may also take place, as is seen following repeated injections of erythrogenic toxins or M-protein. Antistreptococcal antibodies cross-reactive with host tissues may initiate autoimmune phenomena, especially in the presence of complement. Fixation of certain streptococcal antigens to tissue cells may also occur and lead to passive immunological injury.

It is also likely that lymphocytes are activated by streptococcal products, especially at the sites of infection, with increased chances of mutation and activation of "forbidden clones" with autoimmune activity (144). A variant of this possibility is that lymphocytes transformed into blast cells by a streptococcus mitogen (145, 146) might damage the host's tissues, analogous to the damage of syngeneic cells brought about *in vitro* by lymphocytes under the influence of nonspecific transforming agents. Treatment of animals with penicillin facilitates the formation of L-forms which cause carditis in monkeys. Persistence of L-forms, and their reversion *in vivo* to the typical bacterial characteristics, may also contribute to prolonged host-parasite interaction.

The persistence of streptococcal elements in tissues, and the ensuing immune reactions mediated by circulating and cell-bound antibodies, are probably responsible for some of the tissue alterations seen in poststreptococcal infections in human beings, as well as for some of the aspects of acute disease. It is tempting to speculate that individuals who either lack adequate enzyme systems for degrading streptococcal cell walls, or who develop exaggerated immune responses of a certain type to streptococcal antigens, may be predisposed to severe and lasting damage following contact with these bacteria.

In what way are Group A streptococci unique in their association with the development of postinfectious complications? There is a clear relationship between the chemical nature and the biological properties of cellular and extracellular components of different streptococcal groups. Groups A and C share common antigens which cross-react with human heart, and both groups synthesize large amounts of SLO, SLS, SK, hyaluronidase, cell SF and nucleases. The products of these two groups are probably immunologically identical. It is also true that certain cell-wall moieties of many streptococcal groups induce chronic nodules in the connective tissue of rabbit skin, and can persist for long periods in inflammatory foci. Bacterial sonicates can cause myocardial and hepatic lesions indistinguishable from those brought about by Group A streptococci. Nonetheless, outbreaks of rheumatic fever, arthritis or nephritis have not been described in patients infected with Group C or G bacteria. It is, therefore, the following factors associated with Group A streptococci which may explain their unique pathogenetic potential for man: 1) type-specific M-protein antigen, associated with virulence and with nephritis; 2) NAD-glycohydrolase, associated with leukotoxicity; and 3) erythrogenic toxins of scarlet fever. In addition, certain group A strains possess a membrane-associated antigen which cross-reacts with human kidney and which has been implicated in the pathogenesis of AGN.

It would thus appear likely that further research on the specific pathogenic properties of the special group A factors will increase our understanding of the mode of pathogenicity of group A streptococci in man. The major obstacle to progress in this direction remains the fact that the usual laboratory animals exposed to these specific factors do not develop tissue changes similar to those of human lesions. New experimental models of the streptococcal-human host relationship may have to be sought, or reliance may have to be placed on further circumstantial evidence. Our present knowledge of the mechanisms of streptococcal disease in man, and especially of its chronic complications, is still far too limited to permit the formulation of a unified hypothesis of pathogenicity. The purpose of this essay has therefore been only to present in as integrated a manner as possible the most pertinent information now available, and to point to the experimental approaches and theoretical considerations current today in the study of streptococcal disease.

REFERENCES

1. McCARTY M. The hemolytic streptococci, in: Dubos R and Hirsch JG (Eds), "Bacterial and mycotic infections of man," 4th end. Philadelphia, JB Lippincott Co, 1965, pp 365–391.
2. GINSBURG I and GROSSOWICZ N. Group A hemolytic streptococci. I. A synthetic medium for growth from small inocula. *Proc Soc Exp Biol Med* **96**: 108–112, 1957.
3. KRAUSE RM. Symposium on relationship of structure of micro-organisms to their immunological properties. IV. Antigenic and biochemical composition of hemolytic streptococcal cell walls. *Bacteriol Rev* **27**: 369–380, 1963.
4. McCARTY M and MORSE SI. Cell wall antigens of gram positive bacteria. *Adv Immunol* **4**: 249–286, 1964.
5. GHUYSEN JM. Use of bacteriolytic enzymes in determination of wall structure and their role in cell metabolism. *Bacteriol Rev* **32**: 425–464, 1968.
6. CROMARTIE WJ, SCHWAB JH and CRADDOCK JG. The effect of a toxic cellular component of group A streptococci in connective tissue. *Am J Pathol* **37**: 79–99, 1960.
7. ROTTA J. Biological activity of cellular components of group A streptococci *in vivo*. *Curr Top Microbiol Immunol* **48**: 64–101, 1969.
8. KENDAL FE, HEIDELBERGER M and DAWSON MH. A serologically inactive polysaccharide elaborated by mucoid strains of group A hemolytic streptococcus. *J Biol Chem* **118**: 61–69, 1937.
9. LANCEFIELD RC. Current knowledge of type specific M antigens of group A streptococci. *J Immunol* **89**: 307–313, 1962.
10. ROTHBARD S. Bacteriostatic effect of human sera on group A streptococci. III. Interference with bacteriostatic activity by blockage of the leucocyte. *J Exp Med* **82**: 119, 1945.
11. FOLEY SMJ. Studies on the pathogenicity of group A streptococci. II. The antiphagocytic effects of the M-protein and the capsular gel. *J Exp Med* **110**: 617–628, 1959.
12. STOLLERMAN GH. Nephritogenic and non-nephritogenic streptococci. *J Infect Dis* **120**: 258–263, 1969.
13. HALBERT SP. The use of precipitin analysis in agar for the study of human streptococcal infections. III. The purification of some of the antigens detected by these methods. *J Exp Med* **108**: 386, 1958.

14. CARAVANO R (Ed). "Current research on group A streptococci." Amsterdam, Excerpta Medica Foundation, 1968.
15. TODD EW. The differentiation of two distinct serological varieties of streptolysin, Streptolysin O, and Streptolysin S. *J Pathol Bacteriol* **47**: 423–444, 1938.
16. HALBERT SP. Streptolysin O, in: Montie TC, Kadis S and Ajl SJ (Eds), "Microbial toxins." New York, Academic Press, 1970, v 3, p 69–98.
17. SLADE HD and KNOX GA. Nutrition and the role of reducing agents in the formation of streptolysin O by group A hemolytic streptococcus. *J Bacteriol* **60**: 301, 1950.
18. GINSBURG I. Streptolysin S, in: Montie TC, Kadis S and Ajl (Eds), "Microbial toxins." New York, Academic Press, 1970, v 3, p 99–171.
19. GINSBURG I, BENTWICH ZH and HARRIS TN. Oxygen-stable hemolysins of group A streptococci. III. The relationship of the cell-bound hemolysis to streptolysins *J Exp Med* **121**: 633–646, 1965.
20. KOYOMA J. Biochemical studies on streptolysin S. II. Properties of a polypeptide component and its role in the toxin activity. *J Biochem (Tokyo)* **54**: 146–151, 1963.
21. GINSBURG I and HARRIS TN. Oxygen-stable hemolysins of group A streptococci. IV. Studies on the mechanism of lysis by cell-bound hemolysin of red blood cells and Ehrlich ascites tumor cells. *J Exp Med* **121**: 647–656, 1965.
22. ELIAS N, HELLER M and GINSBURG I. Binding of Streptolysin S to red blood cell ghosts and ghost lipids. *Isr J Med Sci* **2**: 302–309, 1966.
23. BERNHEIMER AW. Cytolytic toxins of bacteria, in: Montie TC, Kadis S and Ajl SJ (Eds), "Microbial toxins." New York, Academic Press, 1970, v 1, p 183–212.
24. HIRSCH JG, BERNHEIMER AW and WEISSMAN G. Motion picture study of the toxic action of streptolysins on leucocytes. *J Exp Med* **118**: 223–228, 1963.
25. WEISSMAN G, KEISER H and BERNHEIMER AW. Studies on lysosomes. III. The effects of Streptolysins O and S on the release of acid hydrolases from the granular fraction of rabbit liver. *J Exp Med* **118**: 205, 1963.
26. HIRSCH JG and CHURCH AG. Studies of phagocytosis of group A streptococci by polymorphonuclear leucocytes *in vitro*. *J Exp Med* **111**: 309–322, 1960.
27. GINSBURG I. Mechanisms of cell and tissue injury induced by group A streptococci. *J Infect Dis* (in press).
28. BARNARD WG and TODD EW. Lesions in the mouse produced by Streptolysins O and S. *J Pathol Bacteriol* **51**: 42, 1940.
29. GINSBURG I, ZEIRI N, ZILBERSTEIN Z, BENTWICH S and LAVI S. Effects of Streptolysin S in rabbits, in: Caravano R (Ed), "Current research on group A streptococci." Amsterdam, Excerpta Medica Foundation, 1968, p 190–191.
30. TAN EM and KAPLAN NH. Renal tubular lesions in mice produced by streptococci in intraperitoneal diffusion chambers: Role of streptolysin S. *J Infect Dis* **110**: 55–62, 1962.
31. WEISSMAN G, BECHER B, WIDERMAN G and BERNHEIMER AW. Studies on lysosomes. VII. Acute and chronic arthritis produced by intraarticular injections of Streptolysin S in rabbits. *Am J Pathol* **46**: 129, 1965.
32. COOK J and FINCHAM WJ. Arthritis produced by intraarticular injections of Streptolysin S in rabbits. *J Pathol Bacteriol* **92**: 461–470, 1966.
33. BERNHEIMER AW and CANTONI GL. The cardiotoxic action of preparations containing oxygen-labile hemolysin of *Streptococcus pyogenes*. I. Increased sensitivity of the isolated frog's heart to repeated application of the toxin. *J Exp Med* **81**: 295, 1945.
34. KELLNER A, BERNHEIMER AW, CARLSON AJ and FREEMAN EB. Loss of myocardial contractability induced in the isolated mammalian heart by Streptolysin O. *J Exp Med* **104**: 301, 1956.

35. REITZ B, PRAGER DJ and FEIGEN GA. An analysis of the toxic actions of purified Streptolysin O on the isolated heart and separate cardiac tissues of the guinea pig. *J Exp Med* **128**: 1901–1924, 1968.
36. PRAGER DJ and FEIGEN GA. Response of the sensitized heart to oxidized and reduced Streptolysin O. *Int Arch Allergy Appl Immunol* **38**: 175–189, 1970.
37. ELLIOT SD and DOLE VP. An inactive precursor of streptococcal proteinase. *J Exp Med* **85**: 305–320, 1947.
38. ELLIOT SD. Streptococcal proteinase, in: McCarty M (Ed) "Streptococcal infections." New York, Columbia University Press, 1954, p 56–64.
39. OGBURN CA, HARRIS TN and HARRIS S. Extracellular antigens in steady-state culture of the hemolytic streptococcus. Production of proteinase at low pH. *J Bacteriol* **76**: 142–151, 1958.
40. ELLIOT SD. A proteolytic enzyme produced by group A streptococci with special reference to its effect on the type specific M antigen. *J Exp Med* **81**: 573–592, 1945.
41. BELETSKAYER LV and BURSHTEIN VA. The effect of proteinase of the streptococcus culture filtrates on metachromatic substance of the connective tissue reactions. *Vopr Med Khim* **11**: 70–73, 1966.
42. KELLNER A and ROBERTSON T. Myocardial necrosis produced in animals by means of crystalline streptococcal proteinase. *J Exp Med* **99**: 495–504, 1954.
43. GINSBURG I. Action of streptococcal hemolysins and proteolytic enzymes on Ehrlich ascites tumor cells. *Br J Exp Pathol* **40**: 417–423, 1959.
44. TILLET WS and GARNER RL. The fibrinolytic activity of hemolytic streptococci. *J Exp Med* **58**: 485, 1933.
45. CHRISTENSEN LR. Streptococcal fibrinolysis. A proteolytic reaction due to a serum enzyme activated by streptococcal fibrinolysin. *J Gen Physiol* **28**: 363, 1945.
46. CHRISTENSEN LR and MACLEOD CM. Proteolytic enzyme of serum, characterization, activation and reaction with inhibitors. *J Gen Physiol* **28**: 559, 1945.
47. LACK CH and ROGERS HJ. Action of plasmin on cartilage. *Nature (Lond)* **182**: 948–949, 1958.
48. RATNOFF OD. Increased vascular permeability induced by human plasmin. *J Infect Dis* **112**: 134–142, 1963.
49. KRASNER RI and JANNACH JR. The streptokinase-plasminogen system. II. Its effect on the development of local streptococcal infections in rabbit skin. *J Infect Dis* **112**: 134, 1963.
50. JANNACH JR and KRASNER RI. The streptokinase-plasminogen system. III. Histopathology of enhanced streptococcal virulence in rabbit skin due to activation of this system. *J Infect Dis* **113**: 77–85, 1963.
51. JANNACH JR and FUERST DE. The effect of human and guinea-pig serum on local streptococcal infection and its relation to the streptokinase-plasminogen system. *J Pathol Bacteriol* **89**: 402–406, 1965.
52. KELLNER A and ROBERTSON T. Selective necrosis of cardiac and skeletal muscle induced experimentally by means of proteolytic enzyme solution given intravenously. *J Exp Med* **99**: 387–404, 1954.
53. RATNOFF O. Some relationships among hemostasis, fibrinolytic phenomena, immunity, and the inflammatory response. *Adv Immunol* **10**: 146–228, 1969.
54. FABER V and ROSENDAL K. Streptococcal hyaluronidase. II. Studies on the production of hyaluronidase and hyaluronic acid by representatives of all types of hemolytic streptococci belonging to group A. *Acta Pathol Microbiol Scand* **35**: 159–164, 1954.
55. DURAN-REYNALS F. Tissue permeability and spreading factor in infections. *Bacteriol Rev* **6**: 197–252, 1942.
56. WARREN GH. The influence of hyaluronidase on the course of experimental infections with certain bacteria and viruses. *Ann NY Acad Sci* **52**: 1157–1165, 1950.

57. RUSSELL BE and SHERWOOD NP. Studies on streptococci. II. The role of hyaluronidase in experimental streptococcal infection. *J Infect Dis* **84**: 81–87, 1949.
58. McCARTY M. The occurrence of nucleases in culture filtrates of group A hemolytic streptococci. *J Exp Med* **88**: 181, 1948.
59. TILLET WS, SHERRY S and CHRISTENSEN LR. Streptococcal deoxyribonuclease: Significance in lysis of purulent exudates and production by strains of hemolytic streptococci. *Proc Soc Exp Biol Med* **66**: 189, 1948.
60. WANNAMAKER LW. Streptococcal deoxyribonuclease, in: Uhr JW (Ed), "The streptococcus, rheumatic fever, and glomerulonephritis." Baltimore, Williams and Wilkins Co, 1964, p 140–165.
61. FIRSHEIN W and ZIMMERMAN EM. *In vitro* and *in vivo* effects of deoxyribonucleic acid degradation products on virulent and avirulent group A streptococci. *J Gen Microbiol* **36**: 237–248, 1964.
62. CARLSON AS, KELLNER A, BERNHEIMER AW and FREEMAN E. A streptococcal enzyme that acts specifically upon diphosphopyridine nucleotide: Characterization of the enzyme and its separation from SLO. *J Exp Med* **106**: 15–26, 1957.
63. CARLSON AS, KELLNER A and BERNHEIMER AW. Selective inhibition by preparations of streptococcal filtrates of the oxidative metabolism of mitochondria produced from rabbit myocardium. *J Exp Med* **104**: 577–587, 1956.
64. BERNHEIMER AW, LAZARIDE PO and WILSON AT. Diphosphopyridine nucleotidase as an extracellular product of streptococcal growth and its possible relationship to leukotoxity. *J Exp Med* **106**: 27–37, 1957.
65. BERNHEIMER AW. Recent studies on streptolysin O and streptococcal diphosphopyridine nucleotidase. *Q Rev Pediatr* **15**: 237–243, 1960.
66. OFEK I, RABINOWITZ-BERGNER S and GINSBURG I. Oxygen-stable hemolysins of group A streptococci. VI. The relation of the leukotoxic factor to Streptolysin S. *J Infect Dis* **122**: 517, 1970.
67. OFEK I, FELDMAN S, BERGNER-RABINOWITZ S and GINSBURG I. Application of enzyme production properties in subtyping of group A streptococci according to the T-type. *Appl Microbiol* **22**: 748, 1971.
68. DICK FD and DICK GH. "Scarlet fever." Chicago, Ill, The Year Book Publishers Inc, 1938.
69. WATSON DW and KIM LB. Erythrogenic toxin, in: Montie TC, Kadis J and Ajl, SJ (Eds), "Microbial toxins." New York, Academic Press, 1970, v 3, p 173–187.
70. KIM YB and WATSON DW. A purified group A streptococcal pyrogenic exotoxin. Physiochemical and biological properties including the enhancement of susceptibility to endotoxin lethal shock. *J Exp Med* **131**: 611–628, 1970.
71. SCHWAB JH, WATSON DW and CROMARTIE WJ. Further studies of group A streptococcal factors with lethal and cardiotoxic properties. *J Infect Dis* **96**: 14–18, 1955.
72. SCHUH V. The pyrogenic effect of scarlet fever toxin. I. Neutralization with antitoxin; the nature of tolerance. *Folia Microbiol (Praha)* **10**: 156–162, 1965.
73. LAWRENCE HS. Transfer factor. *Adv Immunol* **2**: 196–261, 1969.
74. HANNA EE and WATSON DW. Host-parasite relationships among group A streptococci. III. Depression of reticuloendothelial function by streptococcal pyrogenic exotoxins. *J Bacteriol* **89**: 154–158, 1965.
75. GLASER RJ, THOMAS WA, MORSE SI and DARNELL JE. The incidence and pathogenesis of myocarditis in rabbits after group A streptococcal pharyngeal infections. *J Exp Med* **103**: 173–188, 1956.
76. ZEIRI N, BENTWICH Z, BOSS JH, GINSBURG I and HARRIS TN. Organ lesions produced in rabbits by group A streptococci and some of their extracellular products. *Am J Pathol* **51**: 351–371, 1967.

77. Spira G, Zilberstein Z, Harris TN and Ginsburg I. Toxic effects induced in rabbits by extracellular products and sonicates of group A streptococci. Proc Soc Exp Biol Med 127: 1196–1201, 1968.
78. Gazit E, Ginsburg I and Harris TN. Dialyzable form of an extracellular streptococcal toxin causing histopathological and biochemical changes in rabbits. Proc Soc Exp Biol Med 140: 1025–1029, 1972.
79. Johnson JC and Stollerman GH. Nephritogenic streptococci. Annu Rev Med 20: 315–371, 1969.
80. Rammelkamp CH Jr. Concepts of pathogenesis of glomerulonephritis derived from studies in man, in: Uhr JW (Ed), "The streptococcus, rheumatic fever and glomerulonephritis." Baltimore, Williams and Wilkins Co, 1964, p 289–300.
81. Unanue ER and Dixon FJ. Experimental glomerulonephritis: Immunological events and pathogenic mechanisms. Adv Immunol 6: 1–79, 1967.
82. Carpenter CB. Immunological aspects of renal disease. Annu Rev Med 21: 1, 1970.
83. Sharp JT. Production of renal disease in the white mouse with streptococcal infection. Proc Soc Exp Biol Med 104: 428–437, 1960.
84. Hinkle NH, Partin J and Clark D. Nephropathy in mice after exposure to group A type 12 streptococci. J Lab Clin Med 56: 265–276, 1960.
85. Reed, RW and Matheson BH. Experimental nephritis due to type specific streptococci. I. The effect of a single exposure to type 12 streptococci. J Infect Dis 95: 191–201, 1954.
86. Reed RW and Matheson BH. Experimental nephritis due to type specific streptococci. II. Effect of repeated exposure to type 12 streptococci. J Infect Dis 95: 202–212, 1954.
87. Reed RW and Matheson BH Experimental nephritis due to type specific streptococci. IV. The effect of type 12 streptococci in monkeys. J Infect Dis 106: 245–249, 1960.
88. Matheson BH and Reed RW. Experimental nephritis due to type specific streptococci. III. Biological, chemical and physical studies of type 12 nephritogenic substance. J Infect Dis 104: 213–232, 1959.
89. Franklin M, Matheson BH and Reed RW. Experimental nephritis due to type specific streptococci. V. Attempts to use tissue cultures and mice for the assay of nephrotoxic streptococcal polypeptides. Can J Microbiol 15: 543–548, 1969.
90. Holm SE, Johnson J and Zettergnen L. Experimental streptococcal nephritis in rabbits. Acta Pathol Microbiol Scan 69: 417–430, 1967.
91. Maki S, Shimotsuji T, Fujisawa H, Ida H, Yoshida N, Atsumi Y, Miyata A, Seino Y and Nakajima J. Studies on the nephritogenicity of hemolytic streptococci. Med J Osaka Univ 19: 175–227, 1968.
92. Fox EN and Winter NK. Multiple molecular structure of the M-proteins of group A streptococci. Proc Natl Acad Sci USA 54: 1118–1125, 1965.
93. Fox EN, Pachman LM, Wittner MK and Dorfman A. Primary immunization of infants and children with group A streptococcal M-protein. J Infect Dis 120: 598–604, 1969.
94. Kendal FE, Heidelberger M and Dawson MH. A serologically inactive polysaccharide elaborated by mucoid strains of group A hemolytic streptococcus. J Biol Chem 118: 61–69, 1937.
95. Johnson BH and Furrer W. Hyaluronic acid: a required component of beta hemolytic streptococci for infecting mice by aerosol. J Infect Dis 103: 135–141, 1958.
96. Willoughby LS, Ginsburg Y and Watson DW. Host-parasite relationship among group A streptococci. I. Hyaluronic acid production by virulent and avirulent strains. J Bacteriol 87: 1452–1456, 1964.
97. Custod JT, Lytle RI, Johson BH and Frank PF. Interdependence of hyaluronic acid and M-protein in streptococcal infections in mice. Proc Soc Exp Biol Med 103: 751–753, 1960.

98. FOLEY MJ. Studies on the pathogenicity of group A streptococci. II. The antiphagocytic effects of the M-protein and the capsular gel. *J Exp Med* **110**: 617–628, 1959.

99. MAXTED WR. Streptococcal bacteriophage, in: Uhr JW (Ed), "The streptococcus, rheumatic fever and glomerulonephritis." Baltimore, Williams and Wilkins Co, 1964, p. 25–49.

100. ZABRISKIE JB. The role of temperate bacteriophage in the production of erythrogenic toxin by group A streptococci. *J Exp Med* **119**: 761–780, 1966.

101. ZWEIFACH BW, GRANT L and MCCLUSKEY RT (Eds). "The inflammatory process." New York, Academic Press, 1965.

102. AYOUB EM and WHITE JC. Intraphagocytic degradation of group A streptococci: Electron microscopic studies. *J Bacteriol* **98**: 728–736, 1969.

103. AYOUB EM and WANNAMAKER LW. Fate of group A streptococci following phagocytosis. *J Immunol* **99**: 1099–1105, 1967.

104. AYOUB EM and MCCARTY M. Intraphagocytic β-N-acetylglucosaminidase. Properties of the enzyme and its activity on group A streptococcal carbohydrate in comparison with a soil bacillus enzyme. *J Exp Med* **127**: 833, 1968.

105. DUDDING BH and AYOUB EM. Persistence of streptococcal group A antibody in patients with rheumatic valvular disease. *J Exp Med* **128**: 1081–1098, 1968.

106. OHANIAN SH and SCHWAB JH. Persistence of group A streptococcal cell walls related to chronic inflammation of rabbit dermal connective tissue. *J Exp Med* **125**: 1137–1154, 1967.

107. SCHWAB JH and OHANIAN SH. Degradation of streptococcal cell-wall antigens *in vivo*. *J Bacteriol* **94**: 1346, 1967.

108. SCHWAB JH and CROMARTIE WJ. Studies on a toxic cellular component of group A streptococci. *J Bacteriol* **74**: 673–679, 1957.

109. SCHWAB JH, CROMARTIE WJ, OHANIAN SH and CRADDOCK JG. Association of experimental chronic arthritis with the persistence of group A streptococcal cell walls in the articular tissue. *J Bacteriol* **94**: 1728–1735, 1967.

110. CROMARTIE WJ and CRADDOCK JG. Rheumatic-like lesions in mice. *Science* **154**: 285–287, 1966.

111. OHANIAN SH, SCHWAB JH and CROMARTIE WJ. Relation of rheumatic-like cardiac lesions of the mouse to localization of group A streptococcal cell walls. *J Exp Med* **129**: 37–49, 1969.

112. GINSBURG I, LAUFER A and ROSENBERG A. Cardiac lesions produced in the rabbit by the intramyocardial injection of various microorganisms. *Br J Exp Pathol* **41**: 19–23, 1960.

113. GINSBURG I, GALLIS AH, COLE RM and GREEN I. Group A streptococci: Localization in rabbits and guinea pigs following tissue injury. *Science* **166**: 1161–1163, 1969.

114. GINSBURG I and TROST R. Localization of streptococci and titanium dioxide particles in arthritic and hepatic lesions in the rabbit. *J Infect Dis* **123**: 292, 1971.

115. RICH AR and GREGORY JE. Experimental evidence that lesions with the basic characteristics of rheumatic carditis can result from anaphylactic hypersensitivity. *Bull Johns Hopk Hosp* **73**: 239–264, 1943.

116. HARRIS TN and HARRIS S. Agglutination by human sera of erythrocytes incubated with streptococcal culture supernates. *J Bacteriol* **66**: 159, 1953.

117. STEWART FS, STEELE TW and MARTIN WT. The mechanisms involved in the production of red cell panagglutinability by streptococcal cultures. *Immunology* **2**: 285–294, 1959.

118. JACKSON RW and MOSKOWITZ M. Nature of a red cell sensitizing substance from streptococci. *J Bacteriol* **91**: 2205–2209, 1966.

119. DISHON T, FINKEL R, MARCUS Z and GINSBURG I. Cell-sensitizing products of streptococci. *Immunology* **13**: 555–564, 1967.

120. GINSBURG I. Experimental arthritis in rabbits induced by passive immune sensitization to a streptococcal antigen (Abst). *Isr J Med Sci* **7**: 629, 1971.

121. ZABRISKIE JB. Mimetic relationships between group A streptococci and mammalian tissues. *Adv Immunol* **7**: 147–188, 1967.
122. KAPLAN MH. Autoimmunity to heart and its relation to heart diseases. *Progr Allergy* **13**: 408–429, 1969.
123. LANGE CG. Chemistry of cross-reactive fragments of streptococcal cell membrane and human glomerular basement membrane. *Transplant Proc* **1**: 959–963, 1969.
124. GOLDSTEIN I, HALPERN B and HALPERN RL. Immunological relationship between streptococcus A polysaccharide and the structural glycoproteins of heart valve. *Nature (Lond)* **213**: 46, 1967.
125. ZABRISKIE JB, HSU KC and SEGAL BC. Heart-reactive antibody associated with rheumatic fever: Characterization and diagnostic significance. *Clin Exp Immunol* **7**: 147–159, 1970.
126. MARKOWITZ AS, ARMSTRONG SH and KUSHNER DS. Immunological relationship between the rat glomerulus and nephritogenic streptococci. *Nature (Lond)* **187**: 1095–1097, 1960.
127. RAPPAPORT FT, MARKOWITZ AJ, McCLUSKEY RT, HANAOKA T and SHIMADEI T. Induction of renal disease with antisera to group A streptococcal membranes. *Transplant Proc* **1**: 981–984, 1969.
128. DIXON FJ. "The role of antigen-antibody complexes in disease." *Harvey Lect* **A58**: 21–52, 1963.
129. FELDMAN JD. Ultrastructure in immunological processes. *Adv Immunol* **4**: 175, 1964.
130. HERSH EM and BODEY GP. Leucocytic mechanisms in inflammation. *Annu Rev Med* **20**: 105, 1970.
131. LINDBERG LH and VOSTI KL. Elution of glomerular bound antibodies in experimental glomerulonephritis. *Science* **166**: 1032–1033, 1969.
132. VOSTI KL, LINDBERG LH, KOSEK JC and RAFFEL S. Experimental streptococcal glomerulonephritis: Longitudinal study of a laboratory model resembling human acute poststreptococcal glomerulonephritis. *J Infect Dis* **122**: 249–259, 1970.
133. SEGAL BC, ANDRES GA, HSU KC and ZABRISKIE J. Studies on the pathogenesis of acute and progressive glomerulonephritis in man by immunofluorescein and immunoferritin techniques. *Fed Proc* **24**: 100, 1965.
134. GILL F and COLE RM. The fate of a bacterial antigen (streptococcal M-protein) after phagocytosis by macrophages. *J Immunol* **94**: 898–915, 1964.
135. KANTOR F. Fibrinogen precipitation by streptococcal M-protein. I. Identity of the reactants, and stoichiometry of the reaction. *J Exp Med* **121**: 849–859, 1965.
136. KANTOR F. Fibrinogen precipitation by streptococcal M-protein. II. Renal lesions induced by intravenous injection of M-protein into mice and rats. *J Exp Med* **121**: 861–876, 1965.
137. TRESER G, SEMAR M, McVICAR M, FRANKLIN A, TY A, SAGEL I and LANGE K. Antigenic streptococcal components in acute glomerulonephritis. *Science* **163**: 676–677, 1969.
138. GOLDSTEIN I and TRUNG PH. Study of the pathogenic action of group A streptococcal, group polysaccharide, and of sonicated extract of group A streptococcal cell-wall, in: Caravano R (Ed), "Current research on group A streptococcus." Amsterdam, Excerpta Medica Foundation, 1968, p 117–126.
139. COLE RM. The structure of the group A streptococcal cells and its L-forms, in: Caravano R (Ed), "Current research on group A streptococcus." Amsterdam, Exerpta Medica Foundation, 1968, p 5–42.
140. FREIMER EH. Studies on L-forms and protoplasts of group A streptococci. I. Isolation, growth and bacteriological characteristics. *J Exp Med* **110**: 853, 1963.
141. TRUNG PH, SCHMITT-SLOMSKA J and BOUE A. Etudes microscope électronique des premiers stades de l'infection des cultures de cellules diploids

humaines par des formes L du streptocoque du group A. *Pathol Biol* (*Paris*) **16**: 431–437, 1968.

142. SCHMITT-SLOMSKA J, SACQUET E and CARAVANO R. Group A streptococcal L-forms. I. Persistence among inoculated mice. *J Bacteriol* **93**: 451–455, 1967.
143. KAGAN GY. Some aspects of investigation of the pathogenic potentialities of L-forms of bacteria, in: Guze L B (Ed), "Microbial protoplasts, spheroplasts ar.d L-forms." Baltimore, Williams and Wilkins Co, 1968, p 279–292.
144. BURNET FM. "The clonal selection theory of acquired immunity." London, Cambridge University Press, 1959.
145. TARANTA A and UHR JW. Poststreptococcal diseases, in: Samter M (Ed), "Immunological deases." Boston, Little, Brown and Co, Inc, 1971, p 601–617.
146. TARANTA A, CUPPARI G and QUAGLIATA F. Dissociation of hemolytic and lymphocyte transforming activities of Streptolysin S preparations. *J Exp Med* **129**: 605, 1969.

A QUANTITATIVE STUDY OF PHAGOCYTOSIS IN THE SPLEEN OF RATS INFECTED WITH *PLASMODIUM BERGHEI*

AVIVAH ZUCKERMAN, DAN T. SPIRA and NOEMI RON

Department of Protozoology,
Hebrew University–Hadassah Medical School, Jerusalem, Israel

INTRODUCTION

Malaria is still one of the chief killers of mankind, with an annual global mortality rate of close to a million. It is primarily a disease of the circulating erythrocyte, caused by an obligate intracellular parasite of the genus *Plasmodium*. In addition to man, monkeys, rodents, birds and lizards are hosts to specific plasmodia.

It is known that anemia in malaria is incommensurate with parasitemia, and that a large proportion of erythrocytes may be destroyed during infection, even when parasitemia is mild (1). The role of erythrophagocytosis as a factor in the etiology of malarial anemia has been documented (1, 2). The spleen, one of the primary blood filters, largely responsible for the removal from the normal circulation of effete or damaged erythrocytes, is greatly stimulated to erythrophagocytosis in the course of malarial infection. Other primary blood filters, such as the liver and bone marrow, also play a similar if less extensive role. Whether erythrophagocytosis is primarily responsible for the excessive anemia of malaria cannot be determined unless the extent of the phagocytosis is quantitated, if only approximately.

Human plasmodia cannot yet be grown serially *in vitro*, nor can they be maintained in the usual laboratory animals, since they can develop only in certain species of primate, including man. It is therefore fortunate that the immunopathology of the rodent malarias has proved to be closely analogous to that of the human malarias, and that the rodent malarias are conveniently available as research tools (3).

The present study, of which preliminary notes have already been reported (2, 4), attempts to assess both qualitatively and quantitatively the

[79]

phagocytic capacity of the splenic phagocytes of rats infected with *Plasmodium berghei*, in order to gain further insight into the possible role of erythrophagocytosis in the causation of malarial anemia in this host-parasite combination.

MATERIALS AND METHODS

Plasmodium berghei is maintained in the Department of Protozoology by weekly blood passage in outbred white mice.

In this study, young adult outbred rats of the "Sabra" line maintained at the Hebrew University animal stock facility were infected with *P. berghei* from infected rats. A "donor" rat was infected with mouse blood, to serve as a source of homologous inoculum. A standard rat-blood inoculum consisted of 20×10^6 infected rat erythrocytes, i.p.

Tail blood films of infected rats were prepared daily, fixed in absolute methyl alcohol and stained with Giemsa's stain. Parasitized erythrocytes were counted per 10,000 erythrocytes, thus avoiding the use of fractions in analyzing the data as percentages. Cumulative parasite counts (i.e., the sum of the daily parasite counts throughout an infection) were noted, as described by Zuckerman et al. (5). This parameter was devised as a rough estimate of the total amount of circulating plasmodial antigen in the bloodstream throughout a malarial infection. Thus, the cumulative parasite count may be identical for a short but severe attack of malaria and for a milder but more protracted attack.

Erythrocyte counts were performed in a Thoma counting chamber. Counts were done on all rats before experimental manipulation, on the day before an animal was killed, and again on the day it was killed, to determine whether anemia was progressing or regressing at the time of termination of the experiment.

Spleen biopsies consisted of 1 to 2 mm³ of splenic tissue. The spleen was exposed by sterile laparotomy under ether anesthesia, and the abdominal muscles and skin were sutured separately after the biopsied tissue was removed. The tissue sample was teased apart at the end of a slide in a drop of normal rat serum; the film was drawn out as if it were a thin blood film, fixed in methanol, and stained in Giemsa's stain. Similar slides were stained in benzidine-Giemsa, as described by Ralph (6). Following fixation, the slide was first treated for 1.5 min in 10% methanol, then for 1 min in 20% H_2O_2 in 70% methanol, and then stained with Giemsa's stain. The presence of hemoglobin in erythrocytes, reticulocytes and erythroblasts, free or phagocytosed, as well as in erythrocyte fragments, is revealed by this technique.

Rats were killed by an overdose of ether. Spleen volumes were determined by saline displacement at necropsy. A stained preparation was made of a small piece of splenic tissue as described above.

Rats were killed according to a preset, and therefore randomized, schedule at daily intervals between days 1 and 25 following inoculation.

Blood counts were taken and spleen films were prepared from 16 uninfected rats at intervals during the same period, in order to control any variations in blood counts or erythrophagocytosis possibly associated with aging. A total of 90 films from 74 infected rats, and of 22 films from 16 control rats were studied.

Several terms are defined below as employed in this study:

Patency: The period during which parasitized erythrocytes may be demonstrated by standard microscopic examination.

Acute rise of the infection: The period, beginning with the onset of patency, during which parasitemias increase from day to day. Repeated schizogony, which involves cytoplasmic cleavage after a series of nuclear divisions, produces numerous daughter cells, called merozoites. During this period, some of the merozoites of each parasitic generation are scavenged by phagocytes in the blood-filtering organs (spleen, liver, bone marrow), together with cellular debris and malarial pigment. The latter is ferrihematate, a degradation product of the digestion of hemoglobin by a plasmodium.

Crisis: The point of peak parasitemia in an infection curve. This point provides the first parasitological sign that acquired immunity has been added to the innate immune mechanisms present during the acute rise of the infection. The first appearance of demonstrable antiplasmodial antibody generally precedes crisis by a day or two.

Chronic state: Following crisis, acquired and innate immune mechanisms combine to reduce parasitemia to a low but demonstrable level, for a period of variable duration. Erythrophagocytosis, rather than the scavenging phagocytosis of debris, pigment and free parasites, becomes marked.

Latency: Immunity has so far suppressed the infection that parasites can no longer be demonstrated by standard microscopic examination. However, parasites continue to persist in very small numbers and are demonstrable, for example, by the ability of "latent" blood to infect a clean recipient host.

RESULTS

Course of infection. As in former studies on *Plasmodium berghei* in the outbred "Sabra" strain of white rat, infections allowed to run their course in the present series of experiments fell into two groups, designated "high-susceptibility" and "low-susceptibility," with parasitemia peaks above and below 15%, respectively. This division of the rat population has been attributed to the relatively sudden onset of age-associated immunity in young adult animals of this strain (7). Data on the infections of the 73 infected rats studied here are therefore analyzed as two separate populations in Table 1, in Fig. 1 and throughout the study.

Initial body weights and erythrocyte counts were identical, and there were no overt signs whereby the eventual susceptibility-category of a given rat could be predicted. However, after the first few days following inoculation, courses of infection in the two groups diverged sharply, and

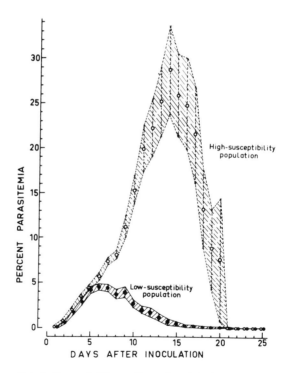

FIG. 1. Course of infection of *Plasmodium berghei,* from inoculation through latency, in rats of "high-" and "low-susceptibility" populations (peak parasitemia above and below 15%, respectively), expressed as mean percent parasitemia ± SE.

TABLE 1. Course of infection in 73 rats infected with Plasmodium berghei, analyzed in two groups

Data	High-susceptibility group: (parasitemia peaks 15% and above)	Low-susceptibility group: (parasitemia peaks below 15%)	Controls
Number of animals at commencement of study	25	48	36
Mean wt in g when inoculated	95.5 ± 2.95	102.0 ± 2.44	98.8 ± 5.30
Mean erythrocyte count × 10⁶/mm³ before inoculation	7.47 ± 0.14	7.51 ± 0.14	7.28 ± 0.12
Mean days prepatent	0.48 ± 0.15	0.79 ± 0.12	—
Mean days of patency in surviving animals reaching latency	17.6 ± 0.86	13.44 ± 0.39	—
Mean peak parasitemia in animals which passed the peak (%)	38.89 ± 4.11 (N = 19)	6.75 ± 0.43 (N = 34)	—
Mean day of peak parasitemia in animals which passed the peak	13.9 ± 0.52 (N = 19)	7.14 ± 0.41 (N = 34)	—
Mortality rate in animals whose infection ran its natural course	4/10 (40.0%)	1/22 (4.5%)	—
Mean day of death	17.5 ± 1.15 (N = 4)	15.0 ± 0 (N = 1)	—
Mean cumulative parasite count in animals dying of parasitemia	25,411 ± 4,885 (N = 4)	1,486 ± 0 (N = 1)	—
Mean cumulative parasite count in animals reaching latency	16,055 ± 2,726 (N = 9)	3,255 ± 305 (N = 28)	—

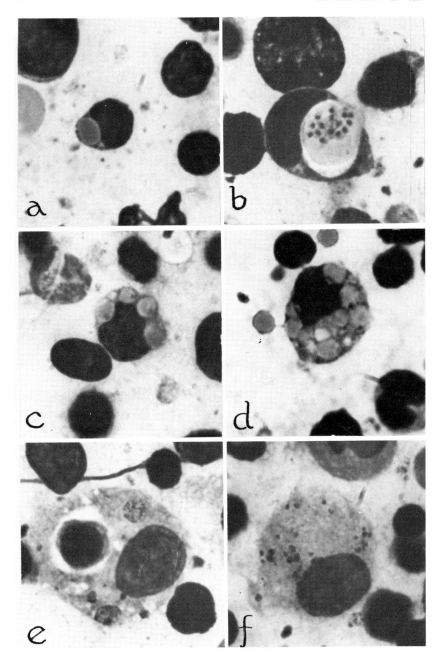

the two groups differed in peak parasitemias, in days of peak, in cumulative parasite counts, in duration of patency and in mortality rates. Since rats were sacrificed at intervals throughout infection and into latency, the "high-susceptibility" population shown in Fig. 1 consisted of 25 rats on days 0, 5 and 10; and of 14, 9 and 7 rats on days 15, 20 and 25, respectively. Similarly, the "low-susceptibility" population consisted of 48, 41, 29, 25, 22 and 19 rats on days 0, 5, 10, 15, 20 and 25, respectively. Since rats were sacrificed on a random basis throughout infection, the number of animals represented in a group varies for the different parameters in Table 1.

The 15% peak parasitemia is merely an empirical boundary demarcating the two very dissimilar populations, whose immune responses do not overlap after the first week. Thus, peak parasitemias of the "high-susceptibility" group in Table 1 had an unstable, broad range, between 15 and 65%, with a 39% mean; while those of the "low-susceptibility" group had a stable and narrow range between 2 and 12%, with a 7% mean.

Forty-nine spleen biopsies were taken from 26 infected rats, one to three times for each rat before it was killed, in order to learn something of the phagocytic activity in the same spleen at different times during the infection course. The operation was well tolerated in all cases. Courses of infection were neither exacerbated nor suppressed by this surgical intervention, but continued without apparent reaction to the surgery,

---

PLATE 1. All photomicrographs are enlarged to the same scale. Whole ingested erythrocytes gradually shrink in the cytoplasm of the phagocyte, but retain their near-spherical contours during early digestion. Parasites remain distinguishable during early digestion. When a digested cell could not longer be defined with confidence, it was registered as "other cell" or, finally, "indeterminate debris."
a) A lymphocyte containing an ingested, unparasitized erythrocyte.
b) A transitional cell ingesting a parasitized erythrocyte. N.B. Reticulocytes, preferentially invaded by *P. berghei*, are more voluminous than definitive normocytes.
c) A transitional cell containing several partially digested erythrocytes, some of digested erythrocytes, three of which are parasitized, and indeterminate debris.
e) A macrophage containing an ingested large lymphocyte, several partially digested which are parasitized, and indeterminate debris.
d) A transitional cell (= a young macrophage) containing numerous partially cells, and indeterminate debris.
f) A macrophage from a rat spleen biopsied during early latency of an infection with *P. berghei*. Only malarial pigment (ferrihematate) is seen in the cytoplasm.

A. ZUCKERMAN ET AL.

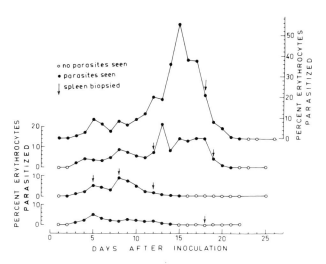

FIG. 2. *P. berghei* infections of varying intensities in rats on which spleen biopsies were performed (↓) at varying stages in the infection course. Note that laparotomy did not appear to disturb the course of infection.

whether the infection was in early patency, at peak, chronic or latent at the time of the operation, or whether it occurred in rats from either the "high-" or the "low-susceptibility" groups (see Fig. 2). Furthermore, phagocytic indexes remained unchanged in the spleens of six control rats biopsied twice to determine whether biopsy stimulated a nonspecific phagocytic reaction. Six additional infected rats were sham-operated. Their spleens were withdrawn from the abdominal cavity, and reintroduced into it without biopsies being taken or the blood vessels severed. The courses of infection of these rats, too, remained uninterrupted by the operation.

Quantitative assessment of phagocytosis in the spleen. Cells in the spleen capable of phagocytosis include all cells in a continuous series from lymphocyte to macrophage. For the sake of convenience in analyzing the results, this series was arbitrarily divided into three categories, lymphocyte, transitional cell and macrophage. This division made it possible to determine whether differentiated macrophages were more efficient phagocytes than the less differentiated precursor cells from which many of them develop in the malarious spleen (8). The position and origin of the various cell types in the splenic architecture are beyond the scope of this study.

PHAGOCYTOSIS IN PLASMODIUM-INFECTED RATS   87

The morphological characteristics of the three categories of phagocyte in Giemsa-stained films are as follows:

a) Lymphocytes: Round cells having spherical or ovoid nuclei with solid blocks of chromatin. The nucleus occupies most of the cell volume. Unvacuolated, basophilic cytoplasm encompasses the nucleus in a narrow rim or half-moon.

b) Transitional cells: Nuclei with kidney-shaped or indented contours, and chromatin progressively more diffuse than in the lymphocyte, but with a chromatin network coarser than that in macrophages. Abundance and basophilia of the cytoplasm intermediate between lymphocytes and macrophages. The cytoplasmic contours tend to be sharp, and the cell borders tend to stain more intensely than the cytoplasm in the interior of the cell.

TABLE 2. *Types of cell and debris ingested by splenic phagocytes of two infected rats. One hundred samples of each of the three types of phagocyte were classified at random in each preparation. Figures represent percentage of phagocytes containing ingested material in each of nine categories. Figures in parentheses represent the mean number of ingested cells observed per positive phagocyte.*

Type of material ingested	Spleen of "low-susceptibility" rat (R79) at 8.6% peak parasitemia, on day 6			Spleen of "high-susceptibility" rat (R35) at 48% peak parasitemia, on day 13		
	Lympho-cytes	Transi-tional cells	Macro-phages	Lympho-cytes	Transi-tional cells	Macro-phages
No phagocytosis	100	87	27	98	89	40
Unparasitized erythrocytes	—	1(1.0)	12(1.4)	—	3	12(1.2)
Unparasitized erythroblasts	—	—	3(1.7)	—	2	33(4.4)
Parasitized erythrocytes	—	—	2(1.5)	—	3	5(1.2)
Parasitized erythroblasts	—	—	—	—	—	—
Other cells	—	—	6(1.2)	—	—	12(2.2)
Erythrocyte fragments	—	1	2	—	—	9
Free parasites	—	—	1	—	—	—
Free pigment	—	10	69	2	5	56
Indeterminate debris	—	3	12	—	—	10

c) Macrophages: Nuclei with a loose and delicate chromatin network and one or more conspicuous nucleoli. The elongate nuclei have irregular contours but their borders are clearly demarcated. The cytoplasm is at least as abundant as the nucleus by volume, and often far more abundant. It tends to contain numerous vacuoles. It takes a pale blue or bluish-grey stain in the body of the cell, and the stain fades by imperceptible degrees towards the cell's irregular and indistinct borders.

Giemsa-stained films of splenic tissue were examined under oil immersion, and 100 randomly-chosen phagocytes of each category were studied. The ingested material in a phagocyte was, of course, not in a uniform state of preservation, since the formed elements had been ingested at different times before fixation, and were therefore in various stages of digestion at the time the film was made.

Each phagocyte was scanned, and its ingested contents were noted under different headings as shown in Table 2, which represents the analysis of two films of splenic tissue from a "high-" and a "low-susceptibility" rat, respectively. Lymphocytes were relatively inefficient phagocytes, and a few phagocytic lymphocytes ingested pigment rather than intact formed cells or cellular debris. As the phagocytes matured, phagocytosis became markedly more intense. A greater proportion of the maturer cells were phagocytic, and each phagocytic cell contained a larger number of a variety of ingested elements, including whole cells and cell fragments. Most of the ingested cells were of the erythroid series. (Anucleate reticulocytes were recorded under "erythrocyte.") "Other cells" included partially digested cells of the erythroid series, which could no longer be assigned with confidence to one of the erythroid categories, as well as occasional clearly defined granulocytes, agranulocytes and even a few macrophages.

The present study is based on 90 such analyses, which include both observations on splenic biopsies and on splenic samples from rats killed at varying stages in the infection. (Not all the samples are represented in each of the analyses below, as some do not fall within the terms of reference of a given summary. Thus, for example, films obtained from an animal killed during patency would not be germane to a summary of data on infections reaching latency.) Together, this material provides a composite record of phagocytic events in the spleens of malarious rats throughout primary infection and into latency. Twenty-two control films from uninfected rats were similarly analyzed.

Phagocytosis by unit numbers of splenic phagocytes throughout primary infection of rats with P. berghei. We first attempted to determine whether individual splenic phagocytes varied in their phagocytic activity throughout the course of infection. Data on "low-" and "high-susceptibility" groups were again analyzed separately. The data in Fig. 3A and B are presented in the form of individual scatter points rather than as statistically analyzed groups, since the number of films available for each day in each group was small, never exceeding six,

Fig. 3A and B record the total number of a) uninfected red cells, with or without nuclei; b) parasitized red cells, with or without nuclei; c) other cells, per 100 lymphocytes, transitional cells and macrophages, respectively, in each available film. Fig. 3A deals with the "high-" and Fig. 3B with the "low-susceptibility" group. Each film is therefore represented in each of the scatter-point diagrams in Fig. 3A and B by a triad of points. The sum of the values of a single triad represents the total number of whole cells contained in 100 splenic phagocytes of a given category for a single film.

Since the "high-" and "low-susceptibility" populations are indistinguishable during the first week of infection (see Fig. 1), all the early data points appear only in the "low-susceptibility" graph, in Fig. 3B.

Mean parasitemias are included in Fig. 3A and B to serve as points of reference for the phagocytic indexes. Standard errors were omitted for simplicity, but were similar to those in Fig. 1. The numbers of spleen samples on which each point in these parasitemia curves is based are recorded in Table 3.

Eighteen films from normal control rats were collected at intervals during infection of the malarious rats. Observations were thus spaced to offset any variations which might occur due to aging. The same 18 samples serve as normal controls in Fig. 3A and B.

The following conclusions may be drawn from Fig. 3A and B:

1) Although phagocytosis by splenic phagocytes in all three categories is stimulated during the infection of rats with *P. berghei,* this stimulation is most extensive in macrophages and least marked in lymphocytes. Thus, lymphocytes are sluggish phagocytes, transitional cells are slightly more reactive and macrophages are far more reactive. In many rats, stimulated macrophages ingested 10 to 30 times as many cells as did normal control macrophages, and in a few rats, macrophages at the height of their phagocytic activity contained as many as 50 times the maximum number of ingested cells found in normal control macrophages. In contrast, stimulated transitional cells never contained more than 10

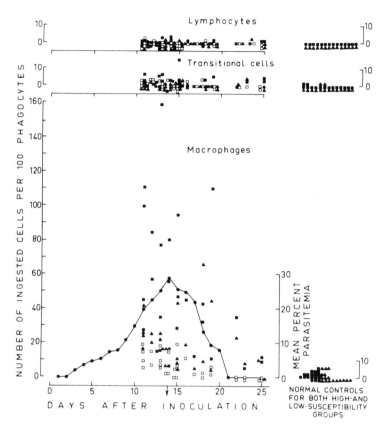

FIG. 3A.   Number of parasitized erythrocytes (□), unparasitized erythrocytes (■)
and other cells (▲) ingested by 100 samples of each of three categories of splenic
phagocyte (macrophages, transitional cells and lymphocytes) in 27 rats of the "high-
susceptibility" group between days 11 and 25 following inoculation, and in 18 normal
control rats. Legend as in Fig. 3B. In order to simplify the graph, mean percent
parasitemias are presented without SE, and all negative phagocytic values appear
below the zero line.

times the maximum number of ingested cells in normal controls, and
stimulated lymphocytes were even less avid. Actually, all ingested cells
observed in lymphocytes represent stimulated phagocytosis, since not one
ingested cell was observed per 100 lymphocytes in any of 18 normal
control films.

2) Thus, the individual splenic phagocyte is on the average a more
efficient ingester of cells and debris at certain times during infection

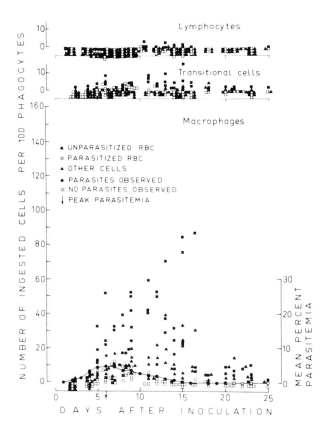

FIG. 3B.   Legend as in Fig. 3A. Normal controls identical with those in Fig. 3A. The population of infected rats consisted of 62 rats of the "low-susceptibility" group between days 2 and 25 following inoculation.

than is its counterpart from an uninfected animal. In macrophages, stimulated phagocytosis of cells occurred between days 5 and 23 in the "low-," and between days 11 (the first recorded day) and 25 in the "high-susceptibility" groups. Thus, stimulated phagocytosis began well wane, into latency. Peak stimulation of phagocytosis fell during the before peak parasitemia in both groups and continued, although on the second week after inoculation in both "high-" and "low-susceptibility" groups. Stimulated phagocytosis in the less avid phagocytes began progressively somewhat later and terminated earlier than in the counterpart macrophages.

TABLE 3. *Number of samples on which the mean percent parasitemias in Fig. 3A and B are based*

Day after inoculation	High-susceptibility group	Low-susceptibility group
1	25	48
2	25	48
3	25	46
4	25	46
5	25	42
6	25	40
7	25	37
8	25	34
9	25	32
10	25	30
11	25	31
12	22	28
13	21	27
14	17	26
15	14	26
16	10	23
17	10	
18	9	24
19	10	24
20	9	23
21	8	23
22	8	23
23	6	5
24		
25	7	19

3) Stimulated phagocytes in all categories ingested significantly more uninfected erythrocytes and erythroblasts than parasitized cells. This was particularly evident at, or near, peak parasitemia, when the spleen is crammed with infected red cells. At this time, moderate phagocytosis of parasitized cells is almost invariably accompanied by very marked phagocytosis of uninfected erythroid cells.

4) Stimulation of splenic phagocytosis was only slightly greater in the "high-" than in the "low-susceptibility" group. This difference was not commensurate with the very marked difference in the severity of the disease observed between the two groups. In fact, the phagocytic responses

of the two groups were in general very similar in nature, in extent and in timing.

Fig. 3A and B represent the ingestion of whole cells by unit numbers of splenic phagocytes. In addition, other formed elements were taken up, and these included parasite pigment (ferrihematate), free parasites, red cell fragments and indeterminate debris in an advanced state of degradation. Data on these were omitted from the figure for simplicity, but are presented in Table 4. Numbers of samples for each day were small (from one to six, with a mean of 3.2). Despite the paucity of the samples, the uptake of each formed element throughout infection proved not to be random, but to follow a relatively stable pattern along the general lines described above for the ingestion of whole cells.

Ingested malarial pigment was a conspicuous feature in a high percentage of phagocytes, particularly macrophages. As expected, pigment accumulated and persisted in many phagocytes into latency.

Few free parasites were observed in phagocytes, although it would seem probable that many such elements must have been cleared from the circulation at every sporulation, since parasitemias rarely became overwhelming and were often very mild. Free parasites may indeed have been taken up frequently, but if they quickly lost their staining properties upon digestion, they would appear under the category of "indeterminate debris." Such debris was indeed more conspicuous in infected rats at and after peak parasitemia than in the controls. However, not all indeterminate debris can originally have been free parasites, since this category of ingested material remained elevated even during latency, when only occasional parasites still persist in the circulation.

Variations in spleen volume and in the total phagocytic potential of the spleen during infection. The total phagocytic load of splenic phagocytes is obviously a function not only of variations in the activity of individual phagocytes, but also in the total number of phagocytes in the spleen. The spleen volumes of 41 infected rats, measured at necropsy by saline displacement, are recorded in Fig. 4. Rats in this study were all of the same age group, and the volumes of nine control rat spleens varied within a narrow range.

At and after day 4 of the infection, spleen volumes first increased and then regressed. This process was directly linked in time and extent with parasitemia courses. Thus, the observed peak of spleen volume in rats of the "low-susceptibility" group (approximately an eightfold increase in volume) occurred on days 8 to 9; while that in the "high-

TABLE 4A. *Formed elements other than whole cells ingested by splenic phagocytes in rats whose erythrophagocytosis is represented in Fig. 3A. Mean percent of each category of phagocyte in which a given formed element was observed on a given day*

		High-susceptibility group, day																								Normal controls
		2	3	4	5	6	7	8	9	10	11	12	13	14	15	16	17	18	19	20	21	22	23	24	25	0
Mean % peak parasitemia		+	2	3	5	6	7	8	11	15	20	23	25	29	26	25	22	13	9	8	+	0	0		0	0
Formed elements ingested																										
Pigment	L										4	5	6	3	8	2	5	3	5			4	2			0
	TC										10	7	9	10	17	5	10	6	10			1	2			5
	M										57	61	50	63	60	62	83	71	73			61	44			28
Free parasites	L										0	0	0	0	+	0	0	0	0			0	0			+
	TC										+	0	+	+	+	0	0	0	0			0	0			0
	M										+	2	+	+	+	0	0	3	1			0	0			0
Erythrocyte fragments	L										+	0	0	0	0	0	0	1	0			0	0			2
	TC										+	0	+	1	2	1	0	+	2			0	0			3
	M										4	3	5	4	3	0	2	4	3			0	0			5
Indeterminate debris	L										+	+	+	0	+	1	0	0	+			3	0			0
	TC										2	3	2	1	4	3	1	0	3			4	1			5
	M										14	18	11	9	14	16	12	21	19			18	11			5

M = macrophages; TC = transitional cells; L = lymphocytes; + = less than 1%.

TABLE 4B. *Formed elements other than whole cells ingested by splenic phagocytes in rats whose erythrophagocytosis is represented in Fig. 3B. Mean percent of each category of phagocyte in which a given formed element was observed on a given day*

		Low-susceptibility group, day																								Normal controls
		2	3	4	5	6	7	8	9	10	11	12	13	14	15	16	17	18	19	20	21	22	23	24	25	25
Mean % peak parasitemia		+	2	3	4	5	4	4	4	3	2	2	1	+	+	+	+	+	+	+	0	0	0	0	0	0
Formed elements ingested																										
Pigment	L	0	0	0	+	5	2	2	5	3	2	1	1	2	2	+	1	1	+	+	0	0	0	0	0	0
	TC	1	1	1	9	16	11	8	9	4	4	+	+	4	6	1	5	5	10	+	0	2	0	+	0	0
	M	2	10	31	37	37	53	55	52	45	51	55	66	65	59	35	56	42	58	56	42	58	34	34	34	25
Free parasites	L	0	0	0	0	0	0	0	+	0	0	0	0	0	0	0	0	0	0	0	0	0	0	0	0	0
	TC	+	+	+	+	0	+	0	+	0	0	0	0	0	0	0	0	0	0	+	0	0	0	0	0	0
	M	0	+	+	2	2	1	+	1	1	2	0	0	0	0	0	0	1	0	0	0	0	0	0	0	0
Erythrocyte fragments	L	0	0	0	0	0	0	+	0	+	+	+	+	+	0	+	+	0	0	0	0	0	0	0	0	0
	TC	0	0	+	+	1	0	1	0	+	2	+	1	0	3	+	+	0	+	+	6	2	+	+	0	+
	M	+	+	2	2	3	1	2	3	2	2	+	2	2	2	2	2	2	+	+	6	5	+	+	1	1
Indeterminate debris	L	0	0	0	0	0	0	0	0	0	+	+	+	+	0	+	0	0	0	0	0	0	0	0	0	0
	TC	+	1	1	2	4	2	2	2	+	2	1	+	+	1	+	+	2	+	+	2	3	+	1	1	+
	M	6	10	13	13	13	14	12	11	11	14	12	19	11	14	14	22	13	34	16	13	16	13	9	9	5

M = macrophages; TC = transitional cells; L = lymphocytes; + = less than 1%.

A. ZUCKERMAN ET AL.

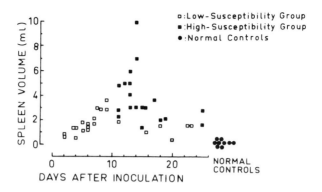

FIG. 4. Spleen volumes of nine normal rats, 22 "low-susceptibility" rats and 19 "high-susceptibility" rats at various stages during infection with *P. berghei*.

susceptibility" group (a mean 17-fold increase in volume) occurred on day 14.

Infections in the "low-susceptibility" group became latent by day 21, and in the "high-susceptibility" group by day 22. Although spleen volumes had regressed appreciably by this time, four out of five spleens were still somewhat enlarged between days 20 and 25.

Quantitative assessment of the increments of different categories of phagocyte appearing as the spleen enlarged was not attempted in this study. Nor were possible nests of ectopic erythropoiesis, such as those observed in the spleens of mice infected with *P. berghei* (9), taken into account. In our experience, such ectopic erythropoiesis may occur, but is not conspicuous in the spleens of infected rats (10).

Spleen volumes therefore aid in roughly assessing the increment in phagocytic function ascribable to the total increase in splenic tissue (see Table 5).

In fact, if anything, the data in Table 5 probably under- rather than overstate the case, for the following reason. Much of the splenomegaly of malaria is attributable to the hypertrophy of macrophages, the dominant phagocyte in the stimulated spleen (8). We have shown that the macrophage is a far more efficient phagocyte than the transitional cell or the lymphocyte, which are relatively less numerous in the stimulated than in the normal spleen. To the extent that the macrophages outnumber the other phagocytes, the total phagocytic capacity would therefore be greater per unit volume of splenic tissue in the stimulated than in the normal spleen. Table 5, however, represents the situation as it would be were there no numerical shift in favor of macrophages during stimulation; and therefore probably represents a conservative rather than an exaggerated estimate. For simplicity, it deals only with the phagocytosis of whole cells, parasitized or unparasitized. The total phagocytic potential would, of course, also include other ingested elements, such as free parasites, pigment, cell fragments and indeterminate debris.

Table 5 presents the values obtained by multiplying the observed number of ingested cells per unit number of phagocytes (as in Fig. 3A and B) by the increment in the splenic volume of each rat, as represented in Fig. 5. The increment was obtained by dividing the observed volume of each infected spleen by the mean volume of nine normal spleens from the same age group of rats ($=0.40 \pm 0.02$ ml).

Deviations from the normal in a) phagocytic activity per unit number of phagocytes, and in b) spleen volume, together contribute to the total phagocytic potential. Since both these parameters are known for each sample in Table 5, the phagocytic potential of each spleen may be calculated for each category of phagocyte. This represents the functional increment of phagocytosis in the given spleen as compared with normal control values. Thus, for example, rat 23 was killed on day 8

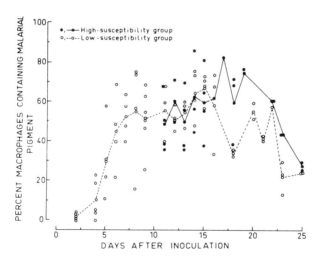

FIG. 5. Accumulation of malarial pigment (ferrihematate) in splenic macrophages of rats infected with *P. berghei*. Each scatter point represents the percentage of such macrophages containing pigment in a single spleen of a rat from the "low-susceptibility" population, and from the "high-susceptibility" population. The graphs represent the daily means of the scatter points for each population.

TABLE 5. *Estimated total phagocytic potential of the spleens of 41 rats at varying stages c normal control rats (see text for definition of parameters). This estimate is based only on th free parasites, ferrihematat*

Rat population	Day when sacrificed following inoculation	No. of rats	Mean spleen volume (ml)	Mean observed volume/ mean control volume
	1	2	3	4
Normal controls	—	9	0.40 ± 0.02	1
Low-susceptibility group	2	2	0.60 ± 0.07	1.50
	4	3	1.10 ± 0.24	2.75
	5	2	1.45 ± 0.25	3.62
	6	3	1.40 ± 0.15	3.50
	7	2	1.90 ± 0.15	4.75
	8	2	2.95 ± 0.04	7.37
	9	2	3.20 ± 0.28	8.00
	11	1	1.80 ± 0.00	4.50
	15	1	1.00 ± 0.00	2.50
	18	1	1.50 ± 0.00	3.75
	20	1	0.40 ± 0.00	1.00
	23	2	1.60 ± 0.00	4.00
High-susceptibility group	11	3	3.30 ± 0.62	8.25
	12	1	5.00 ± 0.00	12.50
	13	4	4.53 ± 0.55	11.32
	14	3	6.67 ± 1.65	16.67
	15	3	2.47 ± 0.44	6.17
	17	1	3.60 ± 0.00	9.00
	18	1	2.00 ± 0.00	5.00
	19	1	2.10 ± 0.00	5.25
	25	2	2.20 ± 0.42	5.50

L = lymphocytes; TC = transitional cells; M = macrophages.

infection with P. berghei *as compared with the phagocytic potential of the spleens of nine uptake of whole blood cells, and ignores other phagocytosed elements (i.e., cell fragments, indeterminate debris).*

5			6			7		
Mean observed number of cells ingested by 100 phagocytes			Mean number of ingested cells in experimental rats/ mean number of ingested cells in control rats			Phagocytic potential of total spleen (value 4 × value 6)		
L	TC	M	L	TC	M	L	TC	M
± 0.00	1.10 ± 0.33	4.90 ± 1.33	0	1	1	0	1	1
0 ± 0.00	1.50 ± 1.06	2.00 ± 0.00	0 : 0	1.37	0.41	0	2.06	0.62
00 ± 0.00	1.33 ± 0.72	5.33 ± 0.27	0 : 0	1.21	1.09	0	3.33	3.00
00 ± 0.00	2.00 ± 0.71	20.00 ± 2.13	0 : 0	1.82	4.08	0	6.59	14.77
00 ± 0.00	8.67 ± 4.38	39.00 ± 15.58	0 : 0	7.88	7.96	0	27.58	27.86
00 ± 0.00	1.50 ± 1.06	9.50 ± 1.06	0 : 0	1.36	1.94	0	7.46	9.22
00 ± 0.00	2.00 ± 0.71	54.00 ± 19.10	0 : 0	1.82	11.02	0	13.41	81.22
0 ± 0.00	3.50 ± 2.48	65.00 ± 4.95	0 : 0	3.18	13.26	0	25.44	106.08
00 ± 0.00	8.00 ± 0.00	56.00 ± 0.00	2 : 0	7.27	11.43	+	32.72	51.44
00 ± 0.00	16.00 ± 0.00	25.00 ± 0.00	1 : 0	14.55	5.10	+	36.38	12.75
0 ± 0.00	6.00 ± 0.00	6.00 ± 0.00	0 : 0	5.45	1.22	0	20.44	4.58
00 ± 0.00	0.00 ± 0.00	9.00 ± 0.00	0 : 0	0.00	1.84	0	0.00	1.84
00 ± 0.00	1.50 ± 1.06	12.00 ± 2.13	0 : 0	1.37	2.45	0	6.48	9.80
00 ± 0.81	2.00 ± 0.94	102.00 ± 25.00	1 : 0	1.82	20.82	+	15.02	171.77
00 ± 0.00	6.00 ± 0.00	90.00 ± 0.00	1 : 0	5.45	18.37	+	68.13	229.63
5 ± 0.65	4.50 ± 1.60	101.75 ± 29.70	0.75 : 0	4.09	20.77	+	46.30	235.12
0 ± 0.47	3.33 ± 1.65	66.33 ± 22.61	1 : 0	3.03	13.54	+	50.51	225.71
3 ± 0.84	7.33 ± 4.35	36.67 ± 11.47	0.33 : 0	6.66	7.48	+	41.09	46.15
0 ± 0.00	0.00 ± 0.00	19.00 ± 0.00	0 : 0	0.00	3.88	0	0.00	34.92
0 ± 0.00	7.00 ± 0.00	6.00 ± 0.00	2 : 0	6.36	1.22	+	31.80	6.10
0 ± 0.00	0.00 ± 0.00	17.00 ± 0.00	0 : 0	0.00	3.47	0	0.00	18.22
0 ± 0.00	3.50 ± 0.35	15.50 ± 2.47	1 : 0	3.18	3.16	+	17.49	17.38

of its infection. Its splenic lymphocytes were not stimulated. However, approximately 20 times as many whole cells were ingested by the total population of splenic transitional cells as by all the transitional cells in a normal rat spleen, and approximately 120 times as many whole cells were ingested by the macrophages of this enlarged spleen as by those of the normal control spleens taken as a group.

The phagocytic potential of the macrophages in infected spleens was significantly increased from day 4 after inoculation through the end of the experiment. Approximately 100-fold stimulation was noted for splenic macrophages in the "low-susceptibility" group on days 8 and 9; and several hundred-fold stimulation in the "high-susceptibility" group between days 11 and 14. After day 14, stimulation of splenic macrophages waned, but remained above normal when the experiment was terminated on day 25.

In general, the phagocytic load of splenic transitional cells followed a similar but less stimulated pattern than that of the macrophages. No stimulation at all was observed for this category of phagocytes in a few animals. Lymphocyets were more frequently stimulated in the "high-susceptibility" group than in the "low." However, in many rats this phagocyte category remained totally quiescent.*

V) *The accumulation of malarial pigment in splenic macrophages in the course of infection with* P. berghei. In malaria, the splenic phagocytes scavenge circulating malarial pigment as a normal aspect of innate immunity: the removal of foreign bodies. Fig. 5 shows that in the malarious rat, most of the macrophages are involved in this function from the second week of infection, and remain so throughout the third week. As of week 4, the percentage of macrophages containing pigment begins to fall, but is still elevated when latency commences (compare with Fig. 1 and 6).

Only macrophages are represented in Fig. 5, but other phagocytes, as well, contained pigment. Throughout the observation period the extent of the pigment burden in lymphocytes and transitional cells stood in

---

* Since the mean phagocytosis for this category was nil in normal rat spleens (see column 5, Table 5), the ratio of "mean observed number of ingested cells" in a stimulated infected spleen to "mean number of ingested cells in normal splenic lymphocytes" (column 6, Table 5) was x:0. Multiplying the values in columns 4 and 6 thus yielded the value 8 for the stimulated lymphocytes in column 7. Since this stimulation, though real, is not high, we chose to designate this value as + rather than 8 in column 7.

approximately the same ratio to the macrophage pigment load as is shown in Fig. 3A and B for the uptake of erythrocytes.

No attempt was made in this study to quantitate the amount of pigment per phagocyte, but it was clear that pigment accumulated in the individual macrophages as the infection progressed. The scavenging of pigment was therefore a continuing process, and the macrophage was shown by its growing pigment burden to be continually phagocytic throughout the study.

No clear distinction was observed between the "high-" and the "low-susceptibility" populations with respect to the uptake of pigment.

VI) *Anemia in the course of infection with* P. berghei. The mean Thoma-cell count of 88 samples of normal rat tail blood from control rats was 7.44 ± 0.07 million erythrocytes per mm³ blood. The erythrocyte count was determined for each infected rat a day or two before inoculation; and generally, two additional counts were made on the day it was killed and on the preceding day. Further counts were not performed, in order to avoid the induction of anemia not due to infection. (The tail blood films required for daily parasitemia counts were obtained by nicking the very tip of the scarred end of the tail. The single drop thus obtained, while serving for a blood film, was insufficient for a red cell count, which requires free bleeding, and which generally involves the loss of numerous drops of blood.)

The 177 available erythrocyte counts of blood samples taken after inoculation were analyzed separately in the two groups defined above, exhibiting "high-" and "low-susceptibility." Daily means ± standard errors in the two groups are compared in Fig. 6 with the normal control group.

As with other parameters, during the first few days of infection the two populations were indistinguishable. Counts on rats presumably of the "high-susceptibility" group, but sacrificed before their parasitemias rose beyond the 15% level, were therefore analyzed with the "low-susceptibility" group. Once anemias of the two populations had diverged, the "high-susceptibility" group was seen to remain more anemic than the "low-susceptibility" group for the duration of the experiment.

Anemias became perceptible by day 4, and were marked by day 7. Peak anemias were reached in the "low-" and the "high-susceptibility" groups on or about days 8 and 16, respectively. In the former group, the recorded blood loss at peak anemia was about a third of the original erythrocyte number; and in the latter, about two thirds.

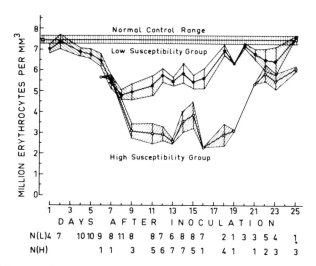

FIG. 6. Mean erythrocyte counts ± SE in 88 normal rat blood samples and in 177 samples from rats during infection with *P. berghei*. The infected blood samples were analyzed in two groups, of "high-" and "low-susceptibility," as defined in the text. N(L), N(H) : number of blood samples in the "low-" and "high-susceptibility" groups, respectively, for a given day.

However, total blood loss was presumably even more extensive than that in the recorded counts, since intense reticulocytosis compensates for the loss of erythrocytes destroyed during malarial infection in rats (11). If this compensatory replenishment of erythrocytes is taken into consideration, Fig. 6 is seen to be, in a sense, the mirror image of Fig. 1, representing parasitemias in the same rats.

Parasitemias reached latency in the "low-" and the "high-susceptibility" populations by days 21 and 22, respectively. Although anemias were waning by this time, blood counts had not yet returned to normal when the parasitemias became latent.

DISCUSSION

Many of the events described here confirm some of the earliest observations in the literature on malarial histopathology and immunology. However, this study differs in one point from most of its predecessors—namely, in the attempt to quantitate observations with regard to both the amount and the character of the phagocytic burden of splenic phagocytes in malarious rats, and the sequence of events relating to parasitemia, splenomegaly, phagocytosis and anemia. Quantitative analysis of erythrophago-cytosis has not hitherto been widely employed, either in general (12) or in malaria in particular, with a few notable exceptions, such as, for example, a study on human malaria by Knüttgen (13).

The excessive anemia of rodent malaria (1, 2, 11, 14–16) is confirmed in the present study, in which recorded anemia was seen to outstrip parasitemia, even though no correction was made here for compensatory reticulocytosis. Thus, 5% peak parasitemias (Fig. 1) were associated with about 30% peak blood loss (Fig. 6); and 30% peak parasitemias with 60% peak blood loss for the "low-" and the "high-susceptibility" groups, respectively. As in former studies (14), excessive anemia was more marked when parasitemias were low than when they were high.

It has long been recognized that, in malaria, blood cells are generally destroyed intracellularly rather than intravascularly, with the exception of blackwater fever (17). As early as 1929, Yorke et al. (18) observed that erythrophagocytosis accompanies intravascular lysis even in extreme cases of blackwater fever. They viewed the two phenomena as graded expressions of the same underlying reaction, a view restated by Davis (19) with respect to malaria in particular and by Bessis and Freixa (20) and Dacie (21) with respect to hemolytic mechanisms in general.

Erythrophagocytosis occurs in malaria in all of the primary blood filter-ing organs but is most prominent in the spleen. Thus, Taliaferro and Mulligan (8) described the spleen as the chief locus in simian malaria, with the liver and bone marrow as important secondary loci. Similar observations have been made on rodent malaria (15, 22) and on avian malaria (23). That erythrophagocytosis plays a central role in the anemia of malaria has repeatedly been pointed out (2, 24, 25). In the present study, attention was therefore focused on the spleen as the primary site of phagocytic activity in malaria, always recalling, however, that all the other sites taken together were probably responsible for at least as much additional phagocytosis as that recorded for the spleen.

It is clear from the present study that, whereas other splenic phago-cytes contribute something to the total phagocytic potential of the malarial rodent's spleen, the lion's share of the phagocytic burden is borne by the macrophage. Although lymphocytes and transitional cells have been analyzed as if they represented distinct categories, all three cell types seem to merge by imperceptible degrees with one another. The evidence for the view that a continuous, interrelated series of cells exists between lymphocytes and macrophages, particularly in the presence of neutrophils or their breakdown products, has recently been reviewed by Pearsall and Weiser (26); this view is supported by the present data, confirming earlier observations on simian malaria (8).

Individual macrophages become increasingly phagocytic as infection progresses, and their phagocytic potential increases following crisis and remains elevated when infections become chronic. Each observed data point, however, obviously represents only an arrested moment in what is an ongoing process in the living cell. Vacuoles, partially digested cells, and indeterminate debris in the macrophage cytoplasm attest to the rapid breakdown of ingested formed elements. Up to 20 ingested and partially digested erythrocytes have frequently been seen in a single macrophage at a given moment. A single such cell could therefore have engulfed literally hundreds of erythrocytes during several weeks of stimulated activity. Actually, the recorded number of ingested erythrocytes is probably too low, since many cells recorded under "other cells" were probably partially digested erythroblasts.

We noted that the erythrocytes in this study were generally ingested as whole cells rather than as fragments. When many erythrocytes are fragmented in the circulation, as by the action of phenylhydrazine (27), the benzidine-positive ingested fragments are clearly distinguishable from whole, even partially digested red cells.

It is noteworthy that we observed few ingested "free parasites." Obviously, not all the merozoites produced invade clean erythrocytes, as attested by the slope of the acute rise of parasitemia curves (Fig. 1). Had all emerging merozoites done so, parasitemia should have been 100% by about day 4, rather than the observed peak of 30% on day 14 in the "high-susceptibility" group. The presumed mechanism of mopping up of circulating merozoites is phagocytosis. Since Giemsa-stained, undegraded, free parasites are readily identifiable, as in thick films of infected blood, and since they were rarely observed in the present study, it would therefore appear that free parasites are probably rapidly degraded on ingestion by splenic phagocytes. If this is true, they probably contribute to the compartment of "indeterminate debris" in our analysis.

Malarial pigment gradually accumulates in splenic phagocytes, as seen in Fig. 5. While the pigment burden of a macrophage can be roughly quantitated (28), this was not done in the present study, where we merely recorded its presence or absence, although we did note that the amount accumulating in a phagocyte increased with time. The source of accumulated pigment could be either a) from parasitized erythrocytes ingested whole, as in Fig. 3A and B; or b) from free pigment scavenged from the circulation, which it reaches when segmenting parasites escape from the host erythrocyte. We cannot assess the relative contributions of these two sources of pigment. Pigment begins to accumulate in splenic macrophages as soon as patency begins, and a large percentage of macrophages contain pigment within a few days. This percentage remains high and relatively stable during the second and third weeks of infection. During the second week, spleen volumes continue to increase and it is reasonable to consider the possibility that some macrophages not containing pigment at this time may be relatively recent arrivals to the blood-filtering compartment (red pulp) of the hypertrophying spleen. That the splenic hyperplasia in malaria is largely associated with the influx of cells of extraneous origin rather than with extensive local mitosis in the red pulp was pointed out by Taliaferro and Mulligan (8).

During the period between days 11 and 16, the "high-" and "low-susceptibility" populations are indistinguishable with respect to the percentage of splenic macrophages containing pigment. From day 16 on, the "high-" appears somewhat to outstrip the "low-susceptibility" group. However, this distinction is doubtful, as it is based on few data points, and may merely reflect the greater duration of patency in the "high-susceptibility" group. After the third week of infection, the number of macrophages containing pigment gradually diminished. This was a somewhat unexpected finding, since ferrihematate has been thought to be a more lasting marker than is suggested by this early downward trend. However, the question of turnover of ferrihematate during late latency was beyond the scope of this study.

An obvious factor influencing the total phagocytic potential of the malarious spleen, in addition to the increased phagocytic activity of the individual macrophage, is the number of macrophages present. Splenomegaly is, of course, one of the chief symptoms of malaria. In this study, as in an earlier one (29), spleen volumes increased and regressed with the kinetics of parasitemia. They peaked on days 9 and 14, for the "low-" and "high-susceptibility" groups, respectively. This timing is practically coincident with peak parasitemia, and comparison of Fig. 1 and 4 strongly suggests that variations in spleen volume are linked with variations in parasitemia. That splenomegaly in malaria fluctuates with overt signs of immunity, including those expressed in the rise and recession of parasitemia, was already stated as a generalization by Taliaferro and Mulligan in 1937 (8). Many authors, including Schofield et al. (8), have noted the direct correlation between splenomegaly and parasitemia in human malaria.

However, whereas spleen volumes in the present study showed a considerable regression by the third week of infection, slight splenomegaly was still apparent, although latency had begun by this time. This is in line with an earlier observation of Ramakrishnan (31), who recorded some splenomegaly in malarious rats even three months after radical cure, confirming our own earlier observations (29). The largest spleens recorded in the present study were about 20 times the normal volume, as compared with about 10 times the normal in other studies on rats with *P. berghei* (31, 32) and three times the normal in monkeys with *Plasmodium knowlesi* (8).

Splenomegaly also develops and regresses at, or after, clinical recovery in other chronic infections, such as tuberculosis, mononucleosis, infectious hepatitis and psittacosis. The phenomenon is associated, in these diseases, as in malaria (1), with anemia due to red cell destruction and stimulation of the reticuloendothelial system (33, 34).

Splenic enlargement in malarious rats is largely due to histiocytic hyperplasia and not, as in malarious mice (9, 35), to ectopic erythropoiesis. Thus, Corradetti (36) points out that the chief site of extramedullary erythropoiesis in the rat is in the liver, with only insignificant foci of erythropoiesis in the spleen. This has been our own experience as well (2). Histiocytic hyperplasia of the spleen, with augmented function of individual macrophages, also characterizes human malaria (37), simian malaria (8), avian malaria (38) and, in general, diseases associated with acute hemolytic anemia (39). Since histiocytic hyperplasia characterizes the rat spleen in the present study, and since we have seen that the macrophage is far more active than other phagocytes, a unit volume of an enlarged malarious spleen is clearly a more effective phagocytic instrument than a unit volume of an unstimulated, normal spleen for two reasons: because each macrophage is more active and because the proportion of macrophages in the total cell population is higher. Were this the only histological variable, doubling the malarious spleen's volume would more than double its phagocytic potential.

Variations in spleen volume have, however, to be employed with caution in assessing total phagocytic potentials of malarious rat spleens. While the red pulp undoubtedly shifts in the histiocytic direction, thus tending to raise the phagocytic potential per unit volume of spleen, the white pulp also undergoes changes during infection. At some times the germinal centers are more densely populated than at others (J. A. Roberts, personal communication). This factor, together with the presence of any islands of erythropoiesis, would tend somewhat to depress the phagocytic potential per unit volume. The values in Table 5 are therefore to be viewed simply as suggesting trends, which we believe would remain substantially as indicated even after the requisite adjustments were made

It has been suggested (32) that the excessive anemia of rodent malaria may be entirely attributed to what is loosely known as "hypersplenism." This condition has been subject to more than one definition. Thus Jandl et al. (34), reiterating earlier statements, define it as the result of repeated episodes of stasis of erythrocytes in a hypertrophied spleen. Increasing degrees of spherocytosis result, and these authors conclude that the spherocytic red cells are eventually trapped and engulfed by virtue of their spherocytic shape alone. It has been questioned (40) whether splenic stasis alone, without antibodies directed against injured red cells, can lead to hemolytic syndromes. Motulsky et al. (41) point out the difficulty of distinguishing between red cell destruction caused by a normally functioning but greatly enlarged spleen and that in which red cell sensitization by autoantibodies also occurs.

Whether the excessive anemia of malaria can be attributed entirely to hypersplenism *sensu strictu*, or whether it may be due in part to an immune phenomenon is therefore still under debate, and the problem has recently been discussed in detail (29). Our view remains, as previously stated (1–3, 29), that, whereas splenic enlargement per se undoubtedly contributes to malarial anemia, it probably is not the exclusive mechanism for red cell destruction. Doan (42) enunciated a broader definition of hypersplenism than Jandl et al. (34). If Doan's definition is accepted, the debate becomes academic, since he includes an element of autosensitization in one form of hypersplenism, which he defines as follows:

1) Inflammatory histiocytic hyperplasia of the spleen in response to an infectious agent,

2) Increased erythrocyte sequestration and congestion in the hyperplastic spleen, leading to slight alteration of the sequestered erythrocytes.

3) Autosensitization of the altered erythrocytes.

4) Increased erythrophagocytosis of altered erythrocytes in the spleen, both as a scavenging function and as a result of specific sensitization by antibody.

5) Anemia as the net result of the above, if erythrophagocytosis outstrips compensatory erythropoiesis.

A similar explanation of events in malarial hypersplenism was suggested by Fairley in 1940 (43). It may be germane that splenic erythrophagocytosis is in general considered to be an important mechanism for the disposal of antibody-coated cells (21, 44, 45). Greendyke et al. (12) have even gone further, stating that erythrophagocytic systems do not operate in the absence of an opsonizing antibody.

Jerusalem (15) pointed out that hypersplenism *sensu strictu* is not the only cause of excessive anemia in malaria, since erythrophagocytosis is also marked in other reticuloendothelial organs, notably the liver. Similarly, Spira and Zuckerman (46) observed anemia in splenectomized malarious rats as extensive as that in intact rats, and considered that liver phagocytes had taken over some of the phagocytic functions of the extirpated spleen.

Erythrophagocytosis is stimulated in the malarious rat spleen not only at and after crisis, but also for several days before crisis (see Fig. 3A and B). The present study demonstrates clearly that splenic phagocytes in the rat infected with *P. berghei* respond to the entire erythron (and not to infected cells alone) as if it were sensitized. Fig. 3A and B show that throughout infection, whether mild or severe, unparasitized erythrocytes, which constituted the bulk of the erythron, were ingested in much greater numbers than parasitized erythrocytes, and that the ingestion of parasitized erythrocytes broadly followed parasitemia curves. Thus, the phagocytic mechanism did not single out the infected cell for special attention, but was keyed to engulfing whatever red cells were currently available, whether parasitized or not. Obviously, some parasitized cells were destroyed in this process, but phagocytosis was erythrocyte-oriented rather than parasite-oriented. From the earliest to the most recent histopathological studies on malaria, all emphasize the ingestion of uninfected together with infected red cells (reviewed in ref. 1). Fairley, in commenting on a talk by Thomson (47), went so far as to state that erythrophagocytosis in malaria was directed against the corpuscle, and that destruction of the parasite was probably an accidental concomitant. Moreover, uninfected erythrocytes are ingested together with infected erythrocytes in other infections with blood protozoa, such as *Babesia canis* (48) and *Babesia rodhaini* (49).

Since the category "other cells" (solid triangles in Fig. 3A and B) probably consists mainly of partially digested erythroblasts, these should be taken into account in computing the total extent of erythrophagocytosis. The complete tally per rat (represented in Fig. 3A and B as the sum of a triad of data points, including a solid and a blank square and a solid triangle at a given point on the time coordinate), is astonishingly high. In the vicinity of peak parasitemia, it may reach an average of an engulfed erythrocyte in every splenic macrophage at a given moment in time. In an *in vitro* study on chicken macrophages (28), homologous erythrocytes were engulfed and completely digested within hours of being presented to the culture macrophages. Even assuming a somewhat slower digestion time for the metabolically more indolent mammalian cell, the ongoing erythrophagocytic destruction of a significant portion of the erythron is constantly and repeatedly taking place in the spleen of the malarious rat, from a few days after inoculation, throughout infection, into latency.

That erythrophagocytosis is the causative mechanism of the excessive anemia of rat malaria therefore seems obvious. The extent of the phago-cytosis is sufficient to explain the loss of one to two thirds of the erythron, and its timing closely coincides with that of the observed anemia. The arguments and rationale for an immune factor in the excessive anemia of malaria have been reviewed (1–3). As late as 1966, the fact that sensitizing antierythrocytic antibody had not yet been demonstrated was still seen as an obvious lacuna in the chain of proof. This gap has since been filled by the demonstration of a cold autohemagglutinin in the serum of rats during the anemic crisis. This can be eluted from the erythrocytes at this time, can coat and sensitize trypsinized but not untrypsinized normal rat erythrocytes to hemagglutination and is sensitive to the action of mercaptoethanol (50, 51). Similar observations have more recently been made on human malaria (50) as well as on avian malaria (53).

Erythrophagocytosis, anemia and autohemagglutinin production thus all occur simultaneously in rodent malaria, and all wax and wane according to similar rhythms, suggesting that all are interrelated. This circumstantial evidence has further led to the suggestion that autologous erythrocyets might be altered *in vivo* by a plasmodial product, possibly an enzyme (2). It remains to be determined whether such a plasmodial product acting on normal rat erythrocytes can prepare these for coating by the autohemagglutinins capable of sensitizing trypsinized normal erythrocytes to autohemagglutination, and whether the autohemagglutinin, whose titer waxes and wanes with anemia and erythrophagocytosis, indeed functions as an autohemopsonin.

Although it was not a part of the original experimental design, the problem of age immunity intruded itself into this study because the rat population employed was of an age when age-associated immunity begins to become manifest. As a result, the infected, outwardly uniform population divided itself into two distinct and separate subgroups, consisting respectively of rats which already had and which had not yet developed age immunity (i.e., "low-" and "high-susceptibility" groups). One week earlier, the animals were propably all highly susceptible, whereas one week later they might all have reached the condition of low susceptibility.

Age immunity in these *P. berghei*-infected rats was apparently associated with an increase in innate immunity, since the slope of the curves during the acute rise of the infection—when only innate immunity is available—was flatter in the "low-" than in the "high-susceptibility" group (see Fig. 1). There is obviously also an increase in acquired immunity, reflected in lower parasitemia peaks, earlier crises, shorter duration of patency and lower mortality rates in the "low-" than in the "high-susceptibility" group. The rather sharp onset of age immunity to *P. berghei* in rats confirms our earlier studies (7, 11).

With respect to the parameters studied here (anemia, splenomegaly and erythrophagocytosis), the "high-" and "low-susceptibility" groups yielded results very similar in kind, but varying in degree, with the severity of the parasitemia.

A possible basis for this age-related shift in susceptibility may be suggested by the observation that the development of age immunity to *P. berghei* in rats is blocked by the administration of antithymocyte serum before the inoculation of plasmodia (54). This would suggest that age immunity in this host-parasite combination may be cell-mediated. A cell-mediated mechanism of immunity in rodent malaria has indeed been demonstrated by the adoptive transfer of protection via immune lymphoid cells (55) and by the cancellation by antithymocyte serum of the ability to acquire age-associated protection (54).

The known facts are compatible with the relatively late maturation of a cell population responsible for the observed intensification and stabilization of innate immunity to *P. berghei* in the young adult rat. An analogy may perhaps be seen in the development of bactericidal activity, presumably associated with increments in lysosomal enzymes and increasing with the age of the host, in rat peritoneal macrophages initially exposed *in vivo* to salmonellae (56). As in the present study, rats acquiring age immunity to salmonellae appeared to have reached a relatively steady reistance state as compared with the more heterogeneous and less effective responses of the younger animal.

In recapitulation of the results of this and other cited studies, the immune and immunopathological responses of rats to initial infection with *P. berghei* include the following major aspects:

1) Age-associated, innate immunity develops in the young adult rat before exposure to *P. berghei,* reducing the intensity of subsequently induced infection and leading to a relatively uniform, steady state of low susceptibility. Age immunity may be thymocyte-dependent.

2) Acquired immunity, following contact with *P. berghei,* is associated with the appearance of protective antiplasmodial antibody, an IgG immunoglobulin. Its only perceptible effect during initial infection is to delay the onset of patency, but with serial superinfections the titer mounts and in some cases can completely protect (57). A cell-mediated factor apparently contributes to acquired immunity, since immune syngeneic splenocytes effectively protect against challenge with viable plasmodia (55).

3) Erythrophagocytosis is conspicuously stimulated during the period ranging from before crisis through latency. It is erythrocyte- rather than plasmodium-oriented, although some infected erythrocytes are ingested together with large numbers of unparasitized erythrocytes. Since erythrophagocytosis occurs during splenic hypertrophy, hypersplenism undoubtedly contributes to the total number of erythrocytes destroyed by erythrophagocytosis. That the size of the enlarged malarious spleen may not, however, be the exclusive cause of erythrophagocytosis, is suggested by the following observations:

a) The excessive anemia of malaria is no less extensive in splenectomized rats infected with *P. berghei* than in normal controls. In splenectomized animals, phagocytosis in the liver is stimulated.

b) Individual macrophages are more avidly phagocytic at the height of malarial anemia than in normal controls.

c) An autohemagglutinin, acting on trypsinized erythrocytes, is present in the plasma of infected rats during the period of peak anemia, and may be eluted from the circulating erythrocytes at this time, when parasitemia is waning or even negligible. Whether the autohemagglutinin also acts as an autohemopsonin remains to be demonstrated.*

---

* It is possible that circulating erythrocytes are fully sensitized by antibody during infection, since additional infected-rat globulin did not curtail survival of these cells upon their transfer to a normal host (58).

Erythrophagocytosis is so extensive in the malarious rat that much, if not all, of the excessive anemia of rodent malaria may be attributed to it.

SUMMARY

Phagocytosis of formed elements of the blood by random samples of three categories of splenic phagocytes (lymphocytes, transitional cells, macrophages) was studied in stained films from the spleens of normal young adult rats and of rats infected with *Plasmodium berghei* throughout infection and latency. These splenic samples represented an important compartment of the lymphoid-macrophage system, but by no means all compartments of that system which are brought into play in malaria.

Phagocytosis was markedly stimulated at and around parasitemia crisis, regressed as infections became chronic, but remained above normal when latency commenced. The macrophage was by far the most active phagocyte, although the other two categories of phagocyte were also stimulated at the height of macrophage stimulation. Unit numbers of macrophages from simulated malarious rat spleens frequently ingested about 20 times as many cells as the same number of normal rat spleno-cytes, and in some cases their phagocytosis was 50-times normal. Erythroid cells were the chief formed element engulfed, although other blood cells and malarial pigment were also frequently ingested. Of the engulfed erythrocytes, the great majority were uninfected cells.

Spleen volumes rose and regressed with parasitemia. The largest spleen which we observed was 20 times the volume of a normal spleen. Splenomegalies were taken into account in assessing the total phagocytic potential of individual malarious rat spleens, and in comparing this potential with that of normal spleens. In severe infections this total potential at peak stimulation was 100 to several hundred times normal.

Anemia in malarious rats was far more severe than that induced by parasitic destruction of red cells, confirming earlier observations. Erythrophagocytosis of normal as well as infected red cells in the spleen and in other organs of the lymphoid macrophage system is sufficiently extensive reasonably to account for the excessive anemia. Erythrophagocytosis and excessive anemia are parallel processes linked in time and extent.

Possible explanations for the excessive anemia observed in rat malaria include hypersplenism, since the spleen normally removes effete erythro-cytes from the circulation, and the larger the spleen, the more extensive the destruction of erythrocytes. However, the greatest observed splenomegaly was only 20 times the normal, whereas the greatest observed erythrophagocytosis of a stimulated spleen was over 200 times normal. Thus, enhancement of erythrophagocytosis by far outstrips enlargement of the spleen. The entire erythron, including infected and uninfected red cells, behaves as if sensitized. Sensitization of the erythron might explain much, if not all, of the excessive anemia. A discussion is presented as to whether an autohemagglutinin, demonstrated in malarious rats during the period of excessive anemia, might also act as an autohemopsonin.

Supported by grant AI 08100 from the United States Public Health Service.

REFERENCES

1. ZUCKERMAN A. Autoimmunization and other types of indirect damage to host cells as factors in certain protozoan diseases. *Exp Parasitol* **15**: 138–183, 1964.
2. ZUCKERMAN A. Recent studies on factors involved in malarial anemia. *Milit Med* **131** (suppl): 1201–1216, 1966.
3. ZUCKERMAN A. Malaria of lower mammals, in: Jackson G J, Herman R and Singer I (Eds), "Immunity to parasitic animals." New York, Appleton-Century-Crofts, 1970, v. 2, p. 793–829.
4. ZUCKERMAN A, SPIRA D and SCHULMAN N. The phagocytic load of splenic macrophages and their precursor cells in rats infected with *Plasmodium berghei. Proc I Int Congr Parasitol (Rome)*, 1964, p 245.
5. ZUCKERMAN A, HAMBURGER J and SPIRA D. Active immunization of rats with a cell-free extract of the erythrocytic parasites of *Plasmodium berghei. Exp Parasitol* **21**: 84–97, 1967.
6. RALPH PH. The histochemical demonstration of hemoglobin in blood cells and tissue smears. *Stain Technol* **16**: 105–106, 1941.
7. ZUCKERMAN A and YOELI M. Age and sex as factors influencing *Plasmodium berghei* infections in intact and splenectomized rats. *J Infect Dis* **94**: 225–236, 1954.
8. TALIAFERRO WH and MULLIGAN HW. The histopathology of malaria, with special reference to the function and origin of the macrophages in defence. *Indian Med Res Mem* **29**: 1–138, 1937.
9. SINGER I. The cellular reactions to infections with *Plasmodium berghei* in the white mouse. *J Infect Dis* **94**: 241–261, 1954.
10. SPIRA D. Blood loss and replacement in intact and splenectomized rats infected with *Plasmodium berghei.* MSc Thesis, Hebrew University, Jerusalem, 1959.
11. ZUCKERMAN A. Blood loss and replacement in plasmodial infections. I. *Plasmodium berghei* in untreated rats of varying age and in adult rats with erythropoietic mechanisms manipulated before inoculation. *J Infect Dis* **100**: 172–206, 1957.
12. GREENDYKE RM, BRIERTY RE and SWISHER SN. *In vitro* studies in erythrophagocytosis. *Blood* **22**: 295–312, 1963.
13. KNUTTGEN HJ. Das menschliche Knochenmark bei akuten Malariainfektionen. *Z Tropenmed Parasitol* **14**: 423–466, 1963.
14. ZUCKERMAN A. Blood loss and replacement in plasmodial infections. II. *Plasmodium vinckei* in untreated weanling and mature rats. *J Infect Dis* **103**: 205–224, 1958.

114   A. ZUCKERMAN ET AL.

15. JERUSALEM C. Über die Anämiegenese bei der Malariainfektion (*Plasmodium berghei*) von NMRI Mäusen. *Z Tropenmed Parasitol* **15**: 371–385, 1964.
16. KRETSCHMAR W. Parasitendichte und Erythrozytenverlust bei der Malaria (*Plasmodium berghei*) in der Maus. *Z Tropenmed Parasitol* **15**: 386–399, 1964.
17. FAIRLEY NH and BROMFIELD RJ. Laboratory studies in malaria and blackwater fever. I. Malaria. *Trans R Soc Trop Med Hyg* **27**: 289–314, 1933.
18. YORKE W, MURGATROYD F and OWEN DU. Observations on five cases of blackwater fever. *Trans R Soc Trop Med Hyg* **23**: 335–384, 1929.
19. DAVIS LJ. Haemolytic anemias. *Edinb Med J* **50**: 589–616, 1943.
20. BESSIS M and FREIXA P. Etudes sur l'ictère hémolytique expérimental par injection et ingestion d'antisérum. *Rev Hemat* **2**: 114–146, 1947.
21. DACIE JV. Haemolytic mechanisms in health and disease. *Br Med J* **5302**: 429–436, 1962.
22. JERUSALEM C. Histo- und biometrische Untersuchungen zur Frage der Autohaemaggression bei Infektion mit *Plasmodium berghei*. *Ann Soc Belge Med Trop* **45**: 405–418, 1965.
23. MCGHEE RB. Erythrophagocytosis in ducklings injected with malarious plasma, in: "Progress in protozoology," *II Int Cong Protozool* (*Lond*) 1965, p 171.
24. TALIAFERRO WH and CANNON PR. The cellular reactions during primary infections and superinfections of *Plasmodium brasilianum* in Panamanian monkeys. *J Infect Dis* **59**: 72–125, 1936.
25. CANNON PR. Pathologic aspect of human malaria, in: Moulton FR (Ed), "Symposium on human malaria." Am Assoc Adv Sci, 1941, p 214–222.
26. PEARSALL NN and WEISER RS. "The macrophage." Philadelphia, Lea and Febiger, 1970, p 27–30.
27. ZUCKERMAN A and SPIRA D. Blood loss and replacement in plasmodial infections. V. Positive antiglobulin tests in rat anemias due to the rodent malarias (*Plasmodium berghei* and *Plasmodium vinckei*), to cardiac bleeding and to treatment with phenylhydrazine hydrochloride. *J Infect Dis* **108**: 339–348, 1961.
28. ZUCKERMAN A. In vitro opsonic tests with *Plasmodium gallinaceum* and *Plasmodium lophurae*. *J Infect Dis* **77**: 28–59, 1945.
29. ZUCKERMAN A, ABZUG S and BURG R. Anemia in rats with equivalent splenomegalies induced by methyl cellulose and *Plasmodium berghei*. *Milit Med* **134** (suppl): 1084–1099, 1969.
30. SCHOFIELD FD, PARKINSON AD and KELLY A. Changes in hemoglobin values and hepatosplenomegaly produced by control of holoendemic malaria. *Br Med J* **1**: 587–591, 1964.
31. RAMAKRISHNAN SP. Studies on *Plasmodium berghei*. VII. Spleen size in albino mice and rats with blood-induced infections. *Indian J Malariol* **6**: 189–198, 1952.
32. GEORGE JN, STOKES EF, WICKER DJ and CONRAD ME. Studies of the mechanism of hemolysis in experimental medicine. *Milit Med* **131** (suppl): 1217–1224, 1966.
33. ROSENTHAL MC, PISCIOTTA AV, KOMNINOS ZD, GOLDENBERG H and DAMESHEK W. The autoimmune hemolytic anemia of malignant lymphocytic disease. *Blood* **10**: 197–227, 1955.
34. JANDL JH, JACOB HS and DALAND GA. Hypersplenism due to infection. A study of five cases manifesting hemolytic anemia. *N Engl J Med* **264**: 1063–1071, 1961.
35. KRETSCHMAR W and JERUSALEM C. Milz und Malaria. Der Infektionsverlauf (*Plasmodium berghei*) in splenektomierten NMRI Mäusen und seine Deutung anhand der histopathologischen Veränderungen der Milz nichtsplenektomierten Mäuse. *Z Tropenmed Parasitol* **14**: 279–310, 1963.
36. CORRADETTI A. A brief account of some outstanding points on the immuno-

logical course of the infection in rodent malaria. *Ann Ist Super Sanita* **3**: 665–679, 1967.

37. CHARMOT G, RIGAUD JL, ANDRE L and FOUCHET M. Considérations sur l'étiologie des splénomegalies tropicales. *Bull Soc Pathol Exot* **56**: 133–137, 1963.

38. CANNON PR and TALIAFERRO WH. Cellular reactions in infection and super-infection with malaria (*P. cathemerium*). *J Prev Med* **5**: 37–64, 1931.

39. DAMESHEK W and SCHWARTZ SO. Acute hemolytic anemia. *Medicine* **19**: 231–327, 1940.

40. SINGER K and DAMESHEK W. Symptomatic hemolytic anemia. *Ann Intern Med* **15**: 544–561, 1941.

41. MOTULSKY AG, CASSERD F, GIBLETT ER, BROWN GO and FINCH CA. Anemia and the spleen. *N Engl J Med* **259**: 1164–1169, 1215–1218, 1958.

42. DOAN CA. The reticuloendothelial cells in health and disease, in: Halpern B, Benacerraf B and Delafresnaye J F (Eds), "Physiopathology of the reticuloendothelial system, a symposium." Oxford, Blackwell Scientific Publications, 1957, chap 19, p 290.

43. FAIRLEY NH. A peculiar hemolytic hypochromic anemia associated with postmalarial splenomegaly of Banti's type. *Trans R Soc Trop Med Hyg* **34**: 173–186, 1940.

44. BONIN JA and SCHWARTZ L. The combined study of agglutination, hemolysis and erythrophagocytosis, with special reference to acquired hemolytic anemia. *Blood* **9**: 773–788, 1954.

45. MOESCHLIN S VON. Die Autoimmunerkrankungen (Autoaggressionskrankheiten). *Acta Haematol (Basel)* **18**: 13–32, 1957.

46. SPIRA D and ZUCKERMAN A. Blood loss and replacement in plasmodial infections. VI. *Plasmodium berghei* in splenectomized rats. *J Infect Dis* **115**: 337–344, 1965.

47. THOMPSON JG. Immunity in malaria. *Trans R Soc Trop Med Hyg* **26**: 483–514, 1933.

48. MAEGRAITH BG, GILLES HM and DEVAKUL K. Pathological processes in *Babesia canis* infections. *Z Tropenmed Parasitol* **8**: 485–514, 1957.

49. SCHROEDER WF, COX HW and RISTIC M. Erythrophagocytosis and hemagglutinins associated with anemia and recovery from *Babesia rodhaini* infections of rats. *J Parasitol* **51** (Sect 2): 30, 1965.

50. COX HW, SCHROEDER WF and RISTIC M. Hemagglutination and erythrophagocytosis associated with the anemia of *Plasmodium berghei* infections of rats. *J Protozool* **13**: 327–332, 1966.

51. KREIER JP, SHAPIRO H, DILLEY D, SZILVASSY IP and RISTIC M. Autoimmune reactions in rats with *Plasmodium berghei* infection. *Exp Parasitol* **19**: 155–162, 1966.

52. KANO K, McGREGOR IA and MILGROM F. Hemagglutinins in sera of Africans of Gambia. *Proc Soc Exp Biol Med* **129**: 849, 1968.

53. GAUTAM OP, KREIER JP and KREIER RC. Antibody coating on erythrocytes of chickens infected with *Plasmodium gallinaceum*. *Indian J Med Res* **58**: 529–543, 1970.

54. SPIRA D, SILVERMAN P and GAINES C. Antithymocyte serum effects on rat malaria. *Immunology* **19**: 759–766, 1970.

55. STECHSCHULTE DJ. Cell-mediated immunity in rats infected with *Plasmodium bergei*. *Milit Med* **134**: 1147–1152, 1969.

56. READE PC. The development of bactericidal activity in rat peritoneal macrophages. *Aust J Exp Biol Med Sci* **46**: 231–237, 1968.

57. ZUCKERMAN A and GOLENZER J. The passive transfer of protection against *Plasmodium berghei* in rats. *J Parasitol* **56**: 379–380, 1970.

58. KREIER JP and LESTE J. Parasitemia and erythrocyte destruction in *Plasmodium berghei*-infected rats. II. Effect of infected host globulin. *Exp Parasitol* **23**: 198, 1968.

THE ROLE OF TOXINS IN THE PATHOGENESIS OF MICROBIAL DISEASE*

H. SMITH

Department of Microbiology, University of Birmingham, Birmingham, England

To what extent are microbial toxins produced in infection, and to what extent are they responsible for the pathogenesis of infectious disease? Conversely, can some harmful effects of microbial infection be explained by phenomena not involving direct toxicity of microbial products? These questions are discussed mainly in relation to the toxic activities of bacteria, since the production of most known microbial toxins has so far been shown for these microbes. However, if only to emphasize the present lack of knowledge, the toxic activities of viruses, fungi and protozoa are mentioned briefly in the context of some principles laid down for bacteria.

In laboratory cultures many pathogenic bacteria and some other types of microbe produce toxins, compounds which damage cells or constituents of animals or plants *in vitro*, and which may harm intact hosts, with possibly fatal consequences. Some toxins are produced extracellularly, but others are found in the cell wall or intracellularly, and are liberated only after lysis of the microorganisms. Are such microbial toxins produced during infectious disease, and are they responsible for the pathological effects; or, can the latter be caused by phenomena other than direct toxicity of microbial products? These questions are discussed, confining attention to animal disease and using the toxic activities of bacteria as the main examples, since most known microbial toxins have so far been associated with bacteria. The object of the paper is to discuss the relevance of microbial toxins in infectious disease, not to describe their mode of action, which has been done elsewhere (1–4). Since much future research

---

* This paper was the opening lecture of the 1970 Oholo Conference on "Microbial Toxins" held in Israel on 4 to 6 March. More recent advances can be obtained from SMITH H and PEARCE JH. Microbial pathogenicity in man and animals. *Symp Soc Gen Microbiol* **22**: 1, 1972.

will deal with the harmful effects of viral, protozoal and fungal infections, the relevance of toxin production in these infections, now largely a matter of conjecture, is discussed briefly towards the end of the paper.

THE ROLE OF TOXINS IN BACTERIAL PATHOGENICITY

Toxins can take part in two aspects of bacterial pathogenicity. During the early stages of infection, toxins can contribute to bacterial invasion by inactivating host defense mechanisms. Thus, the anthrax toxic complex contributes to resistance of virulent *Bacillus anthracis* to phagocytosis because it is produced extracellularly and inactivates phagocytes (5). Immunity to anthrax is based on antibodies to the toxic complex which stop infection at the early, invasive stage. Similarly, staphylococcal α-toxin kills the leukocytes of some animal species and may therefore contribute to staphylococcal invasion in these species. It is noted, however, that many bacterial compounds inhibit host defense mechanisms without being generally toxic, e.g., the capsular polysaccharides of virulent pneumococci. Such compounds not only contribute to primary bacterial invasion but are often the most important factors involved (6).

The primary role of toxins is in contributing to the harmful and sometimes lethal effects on the host which occur during later stages of disease, after the initial bacterial invasion has been successful. The toxic activities of bacteria in producing these pathological effects of disease can be divided into five categories.

1) *Toxins responsible for noninfectious disease because they are produced outside the host.* Bacteria can produce poisons in foodstuffs. The toxin of *Clostridium botulinum* and the enterotoxin of staphylococci are the main examples of these poisons. The disease that occurs on ingestion of the infected food material is a chemical poisoning comparable to that which follows ingestion of a poisonous plant, fungus or shellfish. It is not an infectious process, but clearly the microbial toxin is responsible for disease.

2) *Toxins of cardinal importance in infectious disease. Clostridium tetani* and *Corynebacterium diphtheriae* produce *in vitro* powerful exotoxins which have been well characterized. These toxins are also produced *in vivo* and are responsible for almost the entire disease syndrome; immunization with toxoid protects against disease (1, 2). Much is known about the biochemical activities of these toxins (2). It is emphasized that most pathogenic bacteria do not produce toxins of this type.

3) *Toxins which are significant, but not the only, factors responsible*

for infectious disease. These toxins are produced *in vivo* and are responsible for some of the pathological effects of infection. However, they are not the sole determinants of disease, and often as much toxin is produced by avirulent as by virulent strains. Injection of the toxin does not always produce all the pathological effects of the disease, and usually immunization with toxoid does not confer solid protection against infection (e.g. the α-toxin of staphylococci and the erythrogenic toxin of streptococci) (1). Whether the α-toxin of *Clostridium welchii* should be included here or in the previous section is still an open question. The experimental evidence for and against it being the lethal factor in gas-gangrene seems equally poised (1, 7, 8). Probably the most important representatives of this class of toxins are the endotoxins of Gram-negative bacteria (9). These endotoxins warrant some discussion because their biological properties are striking, and because they have been studied intensively.

Endotoxins are lipopolysaccharides intimately associated with the cell walls of many different Gram-negative bacteria. Their chemistry is known, especially in relation to serological activity (9). When extracted from cell walls by fairly drastic means (treatment with trichloracetic acid or warm aqueous phenol) and injected into animals they produce toxic manifestations—pyrexia, diarrhea, prostration and death. In some infections, there is little doubt that endotoxins are liberated from the cell wall of the invading bacteria and are responsible for pathological effects, such as pyrexia, leukopenia, shock and death in typhoid fever (10); or pyrexia and shock in brucellosis of man, and abortion in brucellosis of domestic animals (11). On the other hand, factors other than endotoxins undoubtedly contribute to the pathology of many Gram-negative infections, as is clear from the following evidence. First, endotoxins have essentially the same biological properties no matter from which bacterial species they are obtained, yet pathological effects of Gram-negative infections vary enormously. Thus, in dysentery and cholera bacteria remain in the gut and there is much diarrhea, whereas in typhoid fever organisms invade the bloodstream and there is relatively little diarrhea; and in cholera there is much more fluid loss from the gut than in dysentery. Second, endotoxin sometimes fails to be released in significant amounts *in vivo.* Thus, avirulent strains of Gram-negative species, including the *Escherichia coli* of normal gut, contain much endotoxin, yet when growing enterically they do not harm the host. Third, an old experiment, often forgotten, is one in which mice genetically resistant to endotoxin nonetheless succumbed to oral infection with *Salmonella typhimurium* (12).

Factors other than endotoxins which may contribute to the pathological effects of Gram-negative infections are as follows: First, aggressins (6) may promote bacterial invasion of blood and tissues where lysis and liberation of endotoxin and other toxic substances can perhaps occur more readily than on body surfaces. This invasion occurs in typhoid fever and brucellosis, where there is more evidence of pathological damage by endotoxin, rather than in diseases such as cholera and dysentery, where the pathogenic organisms remain in the gut. Compounds which may act in this manner are the Vi antigens of salmonellae, the K antigens of *E. coli* and certain cell wall products from brucellae which inhibit humoral and cellular bactericidins (6). Second, differences in nutritional requirements between bacterial species may influence the occurrence of pathological damage by determining bacterial localization in certain tissues where endotoxin and other factors may be released. The massive growth of brucellae in placentas and other fetal tissues, which leads to abortion in certain domestic animals, is determined by the presence in the susceptible tissues of a growth stimulant for brucellae, erythritol (6). Third, and most important in the context of this discussion, the pathologic effects of some diseases may be due to an extracellular or easily liberated toxin, different from endotoxin, which has little relevance in certain diseases because it is not liberated from the cell wall of the causative organism in significant quantities. This situation seems to occur in infections with *Vibrio cholerae, E. coli* and *Pseudomonas aeruginosa* (see below).

4) *Toxins produced* in vitro *but of unknown importance in disease.* Many substances capable of producing toxic effects related or unrelated to disease syndromes have been isolated from cultures. Some of these products may be laboratory artifacts having no relevance to disease *in vivo* (13). Even if they are formed *in vivo,* the question remains whether they play significant roles in infection. Examples are some of the many enzymic and hemolytic products of staphylococci and streptococci, and possibly the "murine" toxin of *Pasteurella pestis* which kills mice but not guinea pigs although both animals are equally susceptible to death by plague (1, 2, 13).

5) *Toxic effects of bacteria* in vivo *for which relevant toxins have not yet been recognized.* As we shall see later, apart from bacteria few pathogenic microbes have been shown to form toxins responsible for the pathologic effects of infection; and despite intensive study, some important pathogenic bacteria also still fall into this category. Examples are *Streptococcus pneumoniae* and *Mycobacterium tuberculosis* (1, 14).

There are two explanations for an apparent lack of toxins. First, toxins may in fact exist but have yet to be demonstrated. Second, the host may be harmed by means other than direct action of a toxin. For example, in diseases where large bacterial populations accumulate before the host succumbs, the growing bacteria might deplete some tissues of essential nutrients, although the versatility of replacement mechanisms of mammalian hosts makes this improbable. A more likely explanation for host damage in the absence of toxin is the evocation of hypersensitivity reactions by otherwise non-toxic bacterial products (see below).

TOXINS REVEALED BY STUDYING BACTERIA IN MORE
NATURAL ENVIRONMENTS

When bacteria grow in laboratory cultures they may not form all the toxic factors which are produced in an animal during infection because the nutritional conditions for bacterial growth *in vitro* are clearly not the same as those *in vivo*. For this reason, it has been suggested (6, 13, 15) that in dealing with unsolved problems of pathogenicity, the behavior of bacteria *in vivo* should be examined for virulence attributes such as toxins. Once recognized *in vivo*, a toxin might then be reproduced under appropriate conditions *in vitro* for closer investigation of its properties. Any investigations *in vivo* should be made in experimental animals or in biological tests in which aspects of the natural disease are simulated as far as possible. In the past decade, several important toxins have been demonstrated by this approach.

The toxic complex now generally accepted as responsible for death from anthrax was first recognized in the plasma of infected guinea pigs and then reproduced *in vitro*; it comprises three synergistically acting components (6, 15). Another toxin, which might be important in death from plague, was recognized when *P. pestis* obtained from infected guinea pigs was investigated to resolve the following anomaly in previous work: Living virulent *P. pestis* killed both guinea pigs and mice; but a product, "murine" toxin, obtained from cultures *in vitro*, killed only mice. However, an extract of *P. pestis* isolated directly from guinea pigs killed guinea pigs as well as mice. Later, guinea pig toxin was found in *P. pestis* grown *in vitro* and fractionated into two synergistically acting components, both proteins, and unconnected with either the "murine" toxin or endotoxin (16). Whether the guinea pig toxin or the "murine" toxin or both are involved in death of man from plague is unknown.

An enterotoxin of *V. cholerae* has been recognized which appears to be responsible for the fatal loss of fluid from the intestine which occurs in cholera. Unsuccessful attempts had previously been made to implicate in cholera the cell wall endotoxin, a mucinase, and other derivatives of *V. cholerae.* The lack of progress was due to the difficulty in obtaining either an experimental animal or a biological test in which the fluid loss effects of cholera could be simulated. Although mice were killed by intraperitoneal injection of living *V. cholerae* and its endotoxin, in neither case were the typical signs of cholera evident. Recent advances have resulted from the use of biological systems in which the effects of cholera could be simulated; and from examination in these systems of the behavior of living *V. cholerae* before studying its products formed *in vitro.*

First, the gross fluid loss of cholera was produced in ligated rabbit gut preparations by young living cultures of *V. cholerae,* and subsequently by filtrates from such cultures (17, 18). The extracellular or easily liberated enterotoxin was heat labile, neutralized by an antiserum to culture filtrates, and not related to mucinase, hemolysin or endotoxin. This rabbit gut technique has been adopted for titration of cholera enterotoxin (19). Second, signs of cholera were produced when young living *V. cholerae* were introduced through a catheter into the washed stomachs of starved 8 to 12-day-old rabbits (20). Filtrates from young, well aerated cultures of *V. cholerae* in simple media produced similar effects. The active material was heat labile, specifically neutralized by antisera to culture filtrates and not connected with endotoxin. At first the enterotoxin was thought to consist of two components, procholeragens A and B, but later (21) procholeragen A was demonstrated to be the important factor. More recently, mongrel dogs have been used in similar experiments to those in young rabbits, with similar results (22, 23).

Craig (24, 25) used skin tests for edema in rabbits and guinea pigs. Furthermore, he examined the extracellular products of *V. cholerae* growing in the natural host, i.e., in filtrates of rice water stools from human cholera patients. These filtrates produced skin edema, in contrast to filtrates from the stools of patients with diarrhea from causes other than cholera. Filtrates from young aerated cultures of *V. cholerae* also produced the skin edema, again in contrast to similar filtrates from *Shigella* spp., *E. coli* and non-cholera vibrios. Serum of human beings who had survived cholera neutralized the edema-producing activity of filtrates from human stools and of cultures of *V. cholerae*. The skin edema factor was heat labile, unaffected by trypsin and distinct from endotoxin.

Clearly, a toxin(s) of *V. cholerae* associated with the lethal effects of cholera has been recognized; the same enterically active compounds are probably present in all crude preparations. The primary need now is purification of the active materials. Whether the skin-reactive and gut-reactive materials are the same or different is still not clear (23, 26, 27). The enterotoxin appears to promote hypersecretion of the gut secretory cells (28), and since it appears to enter the blood stream (29), it could act systemically as well as locally. Whether addition of enterotoxoid will improve conventional cholera vaccines remains to be seen.

Enteropathogenic strains of *E. coli* have been shown to produce a toxin by the ligated rabbit gut technique. Until recently, the causation of diarrhea and scours in children and domestic animals by certain strains of *E. coli* (13) lacked explanation. However, living cultures of *E. coli* strains isolated from babies with diarrhea have now been found to distend ligated rabbit gut preparations, whereas *E. coli* from healthy children and other sources had no effect. A similar gut-distending action was produced by chloroform-killed suspensions of the active strains, but not by similarly killed suspensions of the other strains (30, 31). The enterotoxic activity of the chloroform-killed suspensions was extremely labile and not connected with endotoxic activity. With regard to *E. coli* infections in domestic animals, dilatation of ligated gut preparations from pigs, lambs and calves reflected the enteropathogenicity of *E. coli* strains for the appropriate animal species (32). However, although there was some cross reactivity, a gut preparation from one animal species may not detect a strain pathogenic for another species. Using appropriate ligated gut preparations, enterotoxin was demonstrated in filtrates from soft agar cultures of enteropathogenic strains of *E. coli,* but not in corresponding filtrates from nonenteropathogenic strains (33). The enterotoxins were extracellular, heat labile and nonlethal for mice. They were unrelated to hemolysins and endotoxin; indeed, three preparations of the latter failed to dilate an appropriate ligated gut preparation. The discovery of the enterotoxin(s) of *E. coli* has recently been confirmed (34, 35).

Studies of *Shigella* spp. in ligated rabbit gut preparations have not proceeded as far as those on *V. cholerae* and *E. coli,* but it seems that *Shigella* infections may take a similar course. Signs of dysentery were produced in gut preparations 12 hr after the introduction of live *Shigella* spp. (36). Only freshly isolated strains induced these effects, and subculture *in vitro* soon destroyed the gut-distending activity. Thus, a toxin different from endotoxin might cause at least part of the enteropathogenic effect in dysentery. However, such a toxin has yet to be demonstrated unequivocally, and hypersensitivity to endotoxin might also play a role in the natural diseases (see below).

P. aeruginosa can infect burns, often with fatal consequences. *In vitro,* it forms endotoxin, a lecithinase, a protease and a hemolysin; but none of these compounds seems to fully explain the effects of infection. Liu (37) compared the toxic activity of extracts from lesions produced in rabbit skin by widespread injections of *P. aeruginosa* with that of filtrates from vigorously shaken cultures of the organism in rabbit serum and in broth. The toxin produced *in vivo* and *in vitro* appeared identical from serological evidence: it killed mice in shock, lowered the blood pressure of rabbits, and appeared distinct from any of the previously described products of *P. aeruginosa,* including the endotoxin.

Attempts to demonstrate the production *in vivo* of a toxin from *Listeria monocytogenes* have so far failed (38). However, in these experiments the organisms were not growing freely in the body fluids and tissues of the mice, as occurs in infection. The organisms were restricted to dialysis sacs and Algire chambers placed in the peritoneal cavity. In both systems, bacterial growth appeared to be relatively limited. Furthermore, with dialysis sacs any influence of large molecular host materials would be missed, and with the free passage of soluble materials allowed by Algire membranes, small amounts of relevant microbial products might have escaped from the chambers to be diluted in host fluids.

THE ROLE OF HYPERSENSITIVITY

IN TOXIC MANIFESTATIONS OF DISEASE

Evocation of hypersensitivity reactions by pathogenic bacteria and their products can have serious and even fatal consequences for the host. This has been shown clearly by the classical work with *M. tuberculosis* (1, 39). Furthermore, skin tests clearly indicate that hypersensitive states occur in many other bacterial diseases as well, such as staphylococcal infections, streptococcal infections, pneumococcal infections, brucellosis, tularemia, glanders, leprosy, Johne's disease and salmonellosis (1, 10). Reactions are usually of the delayed type, indicating that cellular mechanisms are involved, but Arthus-type reactions can also occur, e.g., against bacterial polysaccharides (1). Thus, nontoxic bacterial products may produce harm in many diseases by evoking hypersensitivity reactions. The latter are perhaps more likely in chronic than in acute diseases, and especially where

124   H. SMITH

parasites are intracellular. Cellular reactions (40) could be provoked
from time to time by microbial products liberated from the few surviving
intracellular organisms. However, just as production of a toxin *in vitro*
does not necessarily mean that it is relevant *in vivo*, mere demonstration
of a state of hypersensitivity by a skin test is no proof of the implication
of hypersensitivity reactions in the major pathological aspects of the
disease. More extensive investigations are needed; the main systemic and
local effects of a disease must be simulated by hypersensitivity reactions
evoked in a sensitized host by products of the appropriate microorganism.

Evidence for the implication of hypersensitivity reactions in the pathology of a disease is not easily obtained and is often equivocal; animal
models relevant to natural disease are relatively few. It is even more difficult to identify the particular bacterial products involved. For any one
species, these products are likely to be more numerous than those showing
overt toxicity [e.g., for *Brucella abortus* (41)]. The extensive work on
tuberculosis and rheumatic fever emphasizes the difficulties of obtaining
precise biochemical insight in this area (1, 10). There is little doubt, for
instance, that the pathology of tuberculosis is due largely to hypersensitivity to products of *M. tuberculosis* (1, 39). Hypersensitivity also appears
to play a role in the cardiac and kidney lesions following infection with
streptococci, although the influence of direct toxicity of streptococcal products on the susceptible tissues is still advocated, sometimes with convincing experimental evidence. Thus, Ginsburg and his colleagues (4, 42)
showed that rabbits injected i.v. with extracellular products of streptococci
developed myocardial, muscular and hepatic lesions around which, after
subsequent infection with streptococci, phagocytic cells gathered with their
ingested organisms, leading to the possibility of further damage to the
original lesion by streptococcal products. Despite such work, much evidence is accumulating to suggest that damage to cardiac and glomerular
tissue following streptococcal infection is due to evocation of hypersensitivity to some or all of the following antigens: streptococcal antigens
persisting in these sites, host tissue products altered by reaction with streptococcal products, and host glomerular and heart antigens which are immunologically similar to streptococcal products (10, 43, 44). The role of
hypersensitivity in bacterial diseases other than tuberculosis and rheumatic
fever is less clear, for example in pneumococcal pneumonia (45). It
seems to be involved in some nephritic syndromes and in chronic brucellosis (1, 10). And, although in acute brucellosis of domestic animals
abortion is due to the direct toxicity of endotoxin liberated from brucellae

concentrated in certain fetal tissues (11), in other diseases caused by Gram-negative organisms, endotoxin might act more by provoking hyper-sensitivity reactions than by direct toxic action (1). Thus, some infections of primates and other animals with the endotoxin-containing *Shigella* spp. produce the signs of dysentery only after a second challenge (14).

With the increasing importance of the problem of chronic infectious diseases in medicine, the possibility that auto-allergy may be involved in their pathology should be stressed. The biochemical activities of a parasite may change host products sufficiently for them to evoke a tissue-damaging host response. This seems particularly possible for viruses (see below) and appears to occur also with some bacteria, e.g., streptococci (see above). The difficulties of proving a significant role for auto-allergy in the pathology of an infectious disease are similar to those outlined above for hypersensitivity reactions. As far as the writer knows, the nature of any compound involved in "auto-allergy" during infectious disease has not yet been elucidated.

TOXIC ACTIVITIES OF VIRUSES, FUNGI AND PROTOZOA

Although the harmful and lethal effects of infections with viruses, fungi and protozoa are well known, in most cases toxins which might account for the pathological effects have not been clearly recognized. Information is scanty, but there are indications that in some cases, at least, toxins are responsible for harmful effects, and in others hypersensitivity mechanisms appear to play an important role.

VIRUSES

Viruses can produce cytopathic effects in individual cells both in tissue culture and in disease. The cumulative effect of such cell damage in localized areas of an animal host (e.g., poliomyelitis virus in the motor neurons of the anterior horn) or more widespread (e.g., in pox virus in-fections) can account for many of the pathological effects of virus infec-tions, e.g., paralysis in poliomyelitis and shock in pox virus infections (46).

How do viruses produce cytopathic effects in individual cells? The damaging effects could result from what might be called a passive role on the part of the virus, i.e., cells damaged and disrupted after acting as hosts for virus multiplication. Alternatively, cell damage might occur as a sequel to the "cut off" phenomenon, i.e., cessation of host-cell macromolecular synthesis (47). For some viruses, however, such as poliovirus (48, 49), influenza virus (50), mengovirus (51), Newcastle disease virus (52), and pox viruses (53, 54), there is increasing evidence that the cytopathic effects may occur by a more direct "toxic" action of viral products. The cytopathic effects of these viruses on cells are not merely due to virus growth, because it has been shown, by introducing into cells either inactivated virus or fully infective virus with various viral inhibitors, that cell destruction can occur without the necessity of producing new, infectious virus (48, 49, 53, 54). On the other hand, the cytopathic effects are accompanied by virus-induced protein synthesis, and inhibitors of protein synthesis inhibit the cytopathic effects (53, 54). Support for the fact that virus growth and cytopathic effect need not be closely linked is provided by the observation that virulent strains of some viruses, e.g., Newcastle disease virus (52, 55) and mengovirus (51), induce greater cytopathic effects than avirulent strains. However, the larger plaques produced by the virulent strains appeared to be due to greater cytotoxicity and not to faster growth; the burst population of the virulent strains being lower than that of avirulent strains. Also, viruses can grow and not be cytopathic in some cells (e.g., poliovirus in the cells of the alimentary tract), whereas in others, cytopathic effects accompany the growth of the same agent (e.g., poliovirus in the cells of the spinal cord).

Are the virus-induced proteins which accompany the cytopathic effects cytotoxins? At present this is not known and, apart possibly from the penton of adenovirus (56, 57), no virus cytotoxin has been characterized. To answer the question, Stephen and Birkbeck (58) have advocated a direct approach comparable to that used in bacteriology, namely to isolate virus-induced components from infected cells, to free them from intact virus, and to attempt to produce toxic effects in uninfected cells. This approach will require the design of new techniques for the difficult process of introducing potentially cytotoxic viral products into fresh cells.

If cytotoxins are produced by viruses, how do they act? There could be a direct interference with the functions of the cell, just as diphtheria toxin interferes with protein synthesis (1, 4). On the other hand, the virus product might release autolytic enzymes from the cell's own lysosomes (52, 59). Detailed work in this area would obviously be helped by the characterization of virus cytotoxins.

There is increasing evidence that hypersensitivity reactions play a role in the pathology of virus infections. Certainly, skin reactions indicate that hypersensitive states occur in many virus diseases such as smallpox, mumps, measles and virus encephalitis (10). And, since many viruses appear to incorporate host components into their structure, the possibility of "auto-allergic" phenomena occurring is even greater than in bacterial diseases. Deciding whether evocation of hypersensitivity reactions or direct toxicity is responsible for the main pathological effects of virus diseases is not made easier by the present lack of knowledge of virus toxigenicity. Nevertheless, experimental studies in which pathological effects of virus diseases have been provoked or exacerbated by introducing into an infected host antibody or immune cells, indicate that evocation of hypersensitivity or "auto-allergic" reactions are involved in the pathology of rashes (60), lymphocytic choriomeningitis (61, 62) and viral encephalitis (63).

FUNGI

It is clear that fungi can produce toxins. Highly active compounds such as aflatoxin and sporidesmin have been studied intensively (4, 64) and are undoubtedly the cause of much animal disease. However, these fungal toxins correspond to the first class of bacterial toxins mentioned above, namely, they are produced in foodstuffs outside the animal host and they are important only in noninfectious disease. Most fungal toxins fall into this class.

The role of fungal toxins in infectious disease is less clear. Toxins similar to aflatoxin could be responsible for the effects of infection but have yet to be demonstrated unequivocally (64, 65). Peptidases (66), collagenase (67) and elastase (68) appear to be involved in the toxic action of dermatophytes.

Hypersensitivity occurs in many fungal diseases and probably explains to a large degree the pathology of some fungal skin lesions. The compounds responsible for these hypersensitivities are many, even for one fungus, and ill-defined chemically. The degree to which hypersensitivity is implicated in the main pathology of deep mycoses has been less studied than for the dermatophytes, and is still largely a matter for speculation (65, 69).

PROTOZOA

The gross toxic effects of protozoa on their hosts have been investigated, especially those of *Plasmodium* spp.; thus, for example, the red cell destruction, anemia and shock involving circulatory and renal failure that occurs in malaria (70–72). However, no toxin has yet been recognized as being unequivocally responsible for the main pathological effects of any protozoal disease. A toxic material appears to be present in the blood of animals suffering from malaria, but whether this is a direct product of the malarial parasite has yet to be demonstrated (70). The lytic effects of *Entamoeba* spp. on tissues are known, but the microbial enzymes responsible for them have not been isolated (73); and although toxic products of trypanosomes (74) and toxoplasmas (75) have been investigated, their importance in disease is still not clear. Undoubtedly, hypersensitivity and "auto-allergic" phenomena occur in protozoal infections (70, 71, 76), and in some cases they may be responsible for important pathological effects. For example, antibodies to host antigens changed by red blood cell parasitization may, by opsonization, promote phagocytosis and destruction of red blood cells.

This essay began with two questions. First, are microbial toxins responsible for the pathological effects of infectious disease? The answer is "yes" for certain bacterial diseases and "probably yes" for some diseases produced by viruses, fungi and protozoa, although much remains to be done to establish this fact firmly. Second, can the pathological effects be caused by phenomena other than direct toxicity and microbial products? The answer also appears to be affirmative—by evocation of hypersensitivity and "auto-allergic" mechanisms—but proof here is difficult to obtain, and as yet has been provided for only a few diseases.

REFERENCES

1. DUBOS RJ and HIRSCH JG. "Bacterial and mycotic infections of man," 4th edn. Philadelphia, JB Lippincott Co, 1965.
2. VAN HEYNINGEN WE and ARSECULERATNE SN. Exotoxins. *Annu Rev Microbiol* **18**: 195–216, 1964.
3. SMITH H. The toxic activities of microbes. *Br Med Bull* **25**: 288–292, 1969.
4. KLINGBERG MA and TURNER I. "Microbial toxins," 15th Oholo Biological Conference. Ness-Ziona, Israel Institute for Biological Research, 1970.
5. KEPPIE J, HARRIS-SMITH PW and SMITH H. The chemical basis of the virulence of *Bacillus anthracis*. IX. Its aggressins and their mode of action. *Br J Exp Pathol* **44**: 446–463, 1963.
6. SMITH H. Biochemical challenge of microbial pathogenicity. *Bacteriol Rev* **32**: 164–184, 1968.
7. VAN HEYNINGEN WE. The role of toxins in pathogenicity. *Symp Soc Gen Microbiol* **5**: 17–39, 1955.
8. MCLENNAN JD. The histotoxic clostridial infections of man. *Bacteriol Rev* **26**: 177–276, 1962.
9. LUDERITZ O, STAUB AM and WESTPHAL O. Immunochemistry of O and R antigens of *Salmonella* and related *Enterobacteriaceae*. *Bacteriol Rev* **30**: 192–255, 1966.

10. WILSON GS and MILES AA. "Topley and Wilson's principles of bacteriology and immunity." London, Edward Arnold Ltd, 1964.

11. WILLIAMS AE, KEPPIE J and SMITH H. The chemical basis of the virulence of *Brucella abortus*. III. Foetal erythritol a cause of the localization of *Brucella abortus* in pregnant cows. *Br J Exp Pathol* **43**: 530–537, 1962.

12. HILL AB, HATSWELL JM and TOPLEY WWC. The inheritance of resistance, demonstrated by the development of a strain of mice resistant to experimental inoculation with a bacterial endotoxin. *J Hyg (Camb)* **40**: 538–547, 1940.

13. SMITH H and TAYLOR J. "Microbial behaviour *in vivo* and *in vitro*." Cambridge, The University Press, 1964.

14. WATKINS HMS. Some attributes of virulence in *Shigella*. *Ann NY Acad Sci* **88**: 1167–1186, 1960.

15. SMITH H. The use of bacteria grown *in vivo* for studies on the basis of their pathogenicity. *Annu Rev Microbiol* **12**: 77–102, 1958.

16. STANLEY JL and SMITH H. The chemical basis of the virulence of *Pasteurella pestis*. IV. The components of the guinea pig toxin. *Br J Exp Pathol* **48**: 124–129, 1967.

17. DE SN and CHATTERJE, DN. An experimental study of the mechanism of action of *Vibrio cholerae* on the intestinal mucous membrane. *J Pathol Bacteriol* **66**: 559–562, 1953.

18. DE SN, GHOSE ML and SEN A. Activities of bacteria-free preparations from *Vibrio cholerae*. *J Pathol Bacteriol* **79**: 373–380, 1960.

19. KASAI GJ and BURROWS W. The titration of cholera toxin and antitoxin in the rabbit ileal loop. *J Infect Dis* **116**: 606–614, 1966.

20. FINKELSTEIN RA, NORRIS HT and DATTA NK. Pathogenesis of experimental cholera in infant rabbits. I. Observations of the intraintestinal infection and experimental cholera produced with cell-free products. *J Infect Dis* **114**: 203–216, 1964.

21. FINKELSTEIN RA, ATTHASAMPUNNA P, CHULASAMAYA M and CHARUNMETHEE P. Pathogenesis of experimental cholera: Biologic activities of purified procholeragen A. *J Immunol* **96**: 440–449, 1966.

22. SACK RB, CARPENTER CCJ, STEENBURG RV and PIERCE NF. Experimental cholera. A canine model. *Lancet* 206–207, 1966.

23. SACK RB and CARPENTER CCJ. Experimental canine cholera. II. Production by cell-free culture filtrates of *Vibrio cholerae*. *J Infect Dis* **119**: 151–157, 1969.

24. CRAIG JP. A permeability factor (toxin) found in cholera stools and culture filtrates and its neutralization by convalescent cholera sera. *Nature (Lond)* **207**: 614–616, 1965.

25. CRAIG JP. Preparation of the vascular permeability factor of *Vibrio cholerae*. *J Bacteriol* **92**: 793–795, 1966.

26. LEWIS AC and FREEDMAN BA. Separation of type 2 toxins of *Vibrio cholerae*. *Science* **165**: 808–809, 1969.

27. FINKELSTEIN RA and LOS SPALLUTTO JJ. Pathogenesis of experimental cholera. Preparation and isolation of choleragen and choleragenoid. *J Exp Med* **130**: 185–202, 1969.

28. NORRIS HI, CURRAN PF and SCHULTZ SG. Modification of intestinal secretion in experimental cholera. *J Infect Dis* **119**: 117–125, 1969.

29. VAUGHAN WILLIAMS EM and DOHADWALLA AN. The appearance of a choleragenic agent in the blood of infant rabbits infected intestinally with *Vibrio cholerae* demonstrated by cross circulation. *J Infect Dis* **120**: 658–663, 1969.

30. TAYLOR J and BETTELHEIM KA. The action of chloroform-killed suspensions of enteropathogenic *Escherichia coli* on ligated rabbit-gut segments. *J Gen Microbiol* **42**: 309–313, 1966.

31. TAYLOR J, WILKINS MP and PAYNE JM. Relation of rabbit gut reaction to enteropathogenic *Escherichia coli*. *Br J Exp Pathol* **42**: 43–52, 1961.

32. SMITH HW and HALLS S. Observations by the ligated intestinal segment and oral inoculation methods on *Escherichia coli* infections in pigs, calves, lambs and rabbits. *J Pathol Bacteriol* **93**: 499–529, 1967.
33. SMITH HW and HALLS S. Studies of *Escherichia coli* enterotoxin. *J Pathol Bacteriol* **93**: 531–543, 1967.
34. KOHLER EM. Enterotoxic activity of filtrates of *Escherichia coli* in young pigs. *Am J Vet Res* **29**: 2263–2274, 1969.
35. GYLES CL and BARNUM DA. A heat-labile enterotoxin from strains of *Escherichia coli* enteropathogenic for pigs. *J Infect Dis* **120**: 419–426, 1969.
36. ARM G, FLOYD TM, FABER JE and HAYES JR. Use of ligated segments of rabbit small intestine in experimental shigellosis. *J Bacteriol* **89**: 803–809, 1965.
37. LIU PU. The roles of various fractions of *Pseudomonas aeruginosa* in its pathogenesis. III. Identity of the lethal toxins produced *in vitro* and *in vivo*. *J Infect Dis* **116**: 481–489, 1966.
38. DI CAPUA RA, OSEBOLD JW and STONE KR. Toxicity studies of *Listeria monocytogenes* grown *in vivo*. *Am J Vet Res.* **29**: 2023–2028, 1968.
39. DANNENBERG AM JR. Cellular hypersensitivity and cellular immunity in pathogenesis of tuberculosis: specificity, systemic and local nature and associated macrophage enzymes. *Bacteriol Rev* **32**: 85–106, 1968.
40. COOMBS RRA and SMITH H. The allergic response to immunity, in: Gell PGH and Coombs RRA (Eds) "Clinical aspects of immunology." Oxford, Blackwell Scientific Publications, 1968, p 423–456.
41. SMITH H, KEPPIE J, PEARCE JH and WITT K. The chemical basis of the virulence of *Brucella abortus*. IV. Immunogenic products from *Brucella abortus* grown *in vivo* and *in vitro*. *Br J Exp Pathol* **43**: 538–548, 1962.
42. GINSBURG I, GALLIS HA, COLE RM and GREEN I. Group A streptococci: localization in rabbits and guinea pigs following tissue injury. *Science* **166**: 1161–1163, 1969.
43. GOLDSTEIN I, RIBEYROTTE P, PARLERAS J and HOLPERN B. Isolation from heart valves of glycoproteins which share immunological properties with *Streptococcus haemolyticus* Group A polysaccharide. *Nature (Lond)* **219**: 866–868, 1968.
44. McCARTY M. Streptococci, renal disease and transplantation. *Transplant Proc* **1**: 1032–1035, 1969.
45. HEFFRON R. Pneumonia with special reference to pneumococcus lobar pneumonia. New York, Commonwealth Fund, 1939.
46. SMITH HW and WILSON GS. "Mechanisms of virus infection." London, Academic Press, 1963.
47. MARTIN EM and KERR IM. Virus-induced changes in host-cell macromolecular synthesis. *Symp Soc gen Microbiol* **18**: 15–46, 1968.
48. BABLANIAN R, EGGARS HJ and TAMM I. Studies on the mechanism of poliovirus-induced cell damage. I. The relation between poliovirus-induced metabolic and morphological alterations in cultured cells. *Virology* **26**: 100–113, 1965.
49. BABLANIAN R, EGGARS HJ and TAMM I. Studies on the mechanism of poliovirus-induced cell damage. II. The relation between poliovirus growth and virus-induced morphological changes in cells. *Virology* **26**: 114–121, 1965.
50. SCHOLTISSEK C, BECHT H and DRZENIEK R. Biochemical studies on the cytopathic effect of influenza viruses. *J Gen Virol* **1**: 219–225, 1967.
51. AMAKO K and DALES S. Cytopathology of mengovirus infection. I. Relationship between cellular disintegration and virulence. *Virology* **32**: 184–200, 1967.
52. WATERSON AP, PENNINGTON TH and ALLAN WH. Virulence in Newcastle disease virus. A preliminary study. *Br Med Bull* **23**: 138–143, 1967.
53. BABLANIAN R. The prevention of early vaccinia-virus-induced cytopathic effects by inhibition of protein synthesis. *J Gen Virol* **3**: 51–61, 1968.

54. BABLANIAN R. Studies on the mechanism of vaccinia virus cytopathic effects. Effect of inhibitors of RNA and protein synthesis on early virus-induced cell damage. *J Gen Virol* **6**: 221–230, 1970.
55. BANG FB and LUTTRELL CN. Factors in the pathogenesis of virus diseases. *Adv Virus Res* **8**: 199–244, 1961.
56. GINSBERG HS. Biological and biochemical bases for cell injury by animal viruses. *Fed Proc* **20**: 656–660, 1961.
57. GINSBERG HS, PEREIRA HG, VALENTINE RC and WILCOX WC. A proposed terminology for the adenovirus antigens and viron morphological sub-units. *Virology* **28**: 782–783, 1966.
58. STEPHEN J and BIRKBECK TH. The biochemistry of virus cytotoxicity. *J Gen Microbiol* **59**: xvi, 1969.
59. GUSKEY LE, SMITH PC and WOLFF DA. Patterns of cytopathology and lysosomal enzyme release in polio-virus infected HEp-2 cells treated with either 2-(α-hydroxybenzyl)-benzimidazole or guanidine HCl. *J Gen Virol* **6**: 151–162, 1970.
60. MIMS CA. Pathogenesis of rashes in virus diseases. *Bacteriol Rev* **30**: 739–760, 1966.
61. MIMS CA and TOSOLINI FA. Pathogenesis of lesions in lymphoid tissue of mice infected with lymphocytic choriomeningitis (LCM) virus. *Br J Exp Pathol* **50**: 584–592, 1969.
62. OLDSTONE MBA and DIXON FJ. Pathogenesis of chronic disease associated with persistent lymphocytic choriomeningitis viral infection. II. Relationship of the antilymphocytic choriomeningitis immune response to tissue injury in chronic lymphocytic choriomeningitis disease. *J Exp Med* **131**: 1–19, 1970.
63. WEBB HE and SMITH CEG. Relation of immune response to development of central nervous system lesions in virus infections of man. *Br Med J* **2**: 1179–1181, 1966.
64. WRIGHT DE. Toxins produced by fungi. *Annu Rev Microbiol* **22**: 269–282, 1968.
65. AINSWORTH CG. Pathogenicity of fungi in man and animals. *Symp Soc Gen Microbiol* **5**: 242–262, 1955.
66. CHATTAWAY FW, ELLIS DA and BARLOW AJE. Peptidases of dermatophytes. *J Invest Dermatol* **41**: 31–37, 1963.
67. RIPPON JW and PECK GL. Experimental infection with *Streptomyces madurae* as a function of collagenase. *J Invest Dermatol* **49**: 371–378, 1967.
68. RIPPON JW. Elastase production by ringworm fungi, *Science* **157**: 947, 1967.
69. KONG YM and LEVINE HB. Experimentally induced immunity in the mycoses. *Bacteriol Rev* **31**: 35–53, 1967.
70. GARNHAM PCC. Malaria in animals excluding man. *Adv Parasitol* **5**: 139–204, 1967.
71. HUFF CG. Experimental research in avian malaria. *Adv Parasitol* **1**: 1–65, 1963.
72. MAEGRAITH B. "Pathological processes in malaria and blackwater fever." Oxford, Blackwell Scientific Publications, 1948.
73. HOARE CA and NEAL RA. Host-parasite relations and pathogenesis in infections with *Entamoeba histolytica*. *Symp Soc Gen Microbiol* **5**: 230–241, 1955.
74. LUMSDEN WHR. Biological aspects of trypanosomiasis research. *Adv Parasitol* **3**: 1–57, 1965.
75. JACOBS L. *Toxoplasma* and toxoplasmosis. *Adv Parasitol* **5**: 1–45, 1967.
76. ADLER S. Leishmania. *Adv Parasitol* **2**: 35–96, 1964.

ASPECTS OF THE DEFENSE AGAINST
A LARGE-SIZED PARASITE, THE YEAST,
CRYPTOCOCCUS NEOFORMANS

MOSHE ARONSON and JEHUDITH KLETTER

Department of Cell Biology and Histology, Tel Aviv University Medical School,
Chaim Sheba Medical Center, Tel-Hashomer, Israel

Paradoxically, the very first study designed to establish the importance
of phagocytosis as a defense mechanism did not really demonstrate phagocytosis. Metchnikoff's classical experiment (1), in which he inserted the
thorn of a rose bush under the skin of a sea star larva, revealed the
accumulation of phagocytic cells around the foreign body, but not its
engulfment by them. This observation led to the formulation of the
theory of phagocytosis and innumerable experiments were subsequently
conducted, employing various pathogenic and nonpathogenic bacteria,
viruses and fungi, all generally much smaller than the phagocytic cells.

Certain parasites, particularly helminths and some fungi, which are
much larger than the polymorphonuclear (PMN) and mononuclear phagocytes of the host, are nevertheless also often destroyed in the infected
animal. The participation of active cellular processes and the role of
acquired immunity have been amply documented in various studies on
granulomata formed around the eggs of worms such as *Ascaris suis* and
Schistosoma mansoni (2–5). However, the specific mechanisms by which
destruction of the parasites is effected have not yet been elucidated. A
similarly unsolved question is the related problem of the resorption of
catgut in the body: that is, how the enzymes responsible for the process
reach the foreign material.

In many instances, large foreign particles induce what may be considered a "corresponding" tissue reaction, formation of multinucleated
foreign body giant cells. Here again, the mode of formation of these
structures from their precursors, the monocytes, is not yet clear.

It would be of considerable interest to obtain a better understanding
of the mechanisms involved in these related phenomena and to define

[132]

similarities and dissimilarities in the host's responses to small and large parasites. The present communication summarizes experiments towards this goal conducted in our laboratory over a number of years on the mechanisms of resistance of mice, guinea pigs and rabbits to a large-sized pathogenic yeast, *C. neoformans*.

C. neoformans AS AN EXPERIMENTAL MODEL

C. neoformans is an ubiquitous yeast. It is normally saprophytic and does not as a rule settle on the internal or external body surfaces of animals or human beings. It does not form filaments; it reproduces by budding; it can be grown on synthetic media and it forms a polysaccharide capsule. The dimensions of the capsule can be controlled: thus, under certain conditions, small-sized cells which can readily be phagocytized are obtained, and under other conditions (6) large capsules > 70 μ in diameter, a size much larger than that of the phagocytic cells, are obtained.

C. neoformans is an opportunistic parasite, that is, it is normally saprophytic, but will occasionally attack hosts debilitated by another disease, generally one involving the reticuloendothelial system (RES). Leukemia, Hodgkin's disease and other lymphomas may occasionally be accompanied by cryptococcosis. It has not yet been established whether the growth and dissemination of the yeast are facilitated by the primary disease itself, or also by the immunosuppressive treatment generally given to such patients.

Infections in man, dog, cat, horse and cattle are sporadic and infrequent. The most common source of infective material seems to be pigeon excreta (7), which serve as a nitrogenous nutrient for the yeast. The portal of entry is generally the lung, and the fungus develops either in that organ or in the brain. The histopathological manifestations of the disease vary considerably, from lack of any cellular reaction to the appearance of monocytes, granulomata, and the infiltration of lymphocytes and plasma cells. The cryptococci are found both free and engulfed by phagocytic cells.

Only cellular reactions are thought to occur in cryptococcosis; there is usually no evidence for humoral antibody responses (8). Circulating polysaccharides may possibly combine with formed antibodies and may also cause "immune paralysis" (9), as is the case with the pneumococcal polysaccharides (10). In both instances immunization with a large dose of polysaccharide antigen fails to evoke circulating antibody, whereas minute amounts of antigens are effective. There are no reliable procedures for obtaining immune serum and small-capsule strains are utilized for this purpose experimentally. A recent review aptly sums up the possibilities of diagnostic serology: "The absence of suitable serologic procedures and antigen to demonstrate regular circulating antibodies or dermal hypersensitivity in cryptococcosis continue to be an enigma in the serologic investigation of respiratory mycoses" (11).

The mouse is relatively susceptible to the parasite, while the rabbit is resistant. Contradictory reports have been published on the resistance of guinea pigs (12). Our own strain of guinea pigs proved resistant to C. neoformans, although the yeasts were destroyed more slowly than in the rabbit.

It is often difficult to evaluate the virulence of a particular strain of cryptococcus from the dose response, even in the susceptible mouse (8). In our strains, little difference was noted in the mortality rates following i.p. injections ranging from 10^4 to 10^7 organisms. Some animals died within two weeks, others within a month or two, and still others survived for as long as 6 to 12 months.

FACTORS INVOLVED IN RESISTANCE TO C. neoformans

1) The rabbit is resistant to cryptococcal infection, supposedly because of its high body temperature: 39.5 C (12, 13). 2) The polysaccharide capsule of the yeast inhibits phagocytosis to some extent (14). On the other hand, there is no relation between capsular size and virulence (6). 3) Passive immunization with immune rabbit serum (IRS) prolongs the lifespan of infected mice but does not cure the animals (15). 4) Cationic proteins with anticryptococcal properties have been isolated from rabbit PMN cells (16). 5) Egg-white lysozyme is fungicidal for C. neoformans (16). 6) Sera of various animals inhibit the growth of C. neoformans. The serum factors are not well characterized. Their activity is abolished by the addition of phosphate ions but not by EDTA (17, 18). The interested reader is referred to Littman and Zimmerman (12) and to Al-Doory (19) for extensive bibliographies.

THE RING PHENOMENON: OUTLINE OF THE PRESENT WORK

The basic observations (20) from which the present study developed are the following:

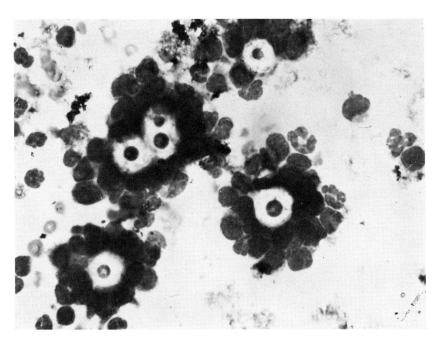

FIG. 1.   Monocyte rings surrounding *C. neoformans* cells. The yeasts were opsonized with moderate amounts of IRS and the smear was made 24 hr after i.p. injection into mice. Note increased basophilia in ring monocytes. Giemsa stain. × 500.

1) Mice were inoculated i.p. with *C. neoformans* together with IRS. Whereas the small cryptococci were phagocytized, the large sized cryptococci became surrounded by rings of monocytes (Fig. 1). In these experiments the rings were two-dimensional; no monocytes settled on top of the surrounded yeasts. The ring monocytes were more basophilic than free monocytes.

2) Neither phagocytosis nor ring formation occurred in the absence of serum.

3) Rings were formed within a few hours of injection, and after several days layers of concentric rings of monocytes of varying thickness were seen around each *C. neoformans* cell. These structures were found on the omentum, onto which most of the injected cryptococci adhered.

These findings raised several questions: a) What is the specific role of immune serum in ring formation? b) Why are the rings two- rather than three-dimensional? c) Are the ring cells capable of destroying the encircled parasite, and if so, by what mechanism? d) Why are ring monocytes more basophilic than free monocytes? Are these cells synthesizing more proteins, involved in destroying the yeast, or are they preparing for mitosis, in which case outer rings might be formed by the division of cells in inner rings? e) The ring structure becomes more complex with time. What is the sequence of cellular responses following the injection of *C. neoformans?* This paper describes studies designed to provide answers to some of these questions.

C. neoformans was maintained and grown on Sabouraud's medium. When larger capsules were required, the yeasts were cultivated on the medium of Littman and Tsubura (6) at 28 C for 7 hr and then for an additional 16 hr at 37 C.

In experiments on inactivation, 3×10^3 yeast cells /ml were incubated for periods of 8 to 72 hr in serum and were then plated on Sabouraud's agar.

Peritoneal cell lysates were prepared by freezing and thawing exudate cells 5 to 10 times. Lysates were similarly prepared from all the formed elements of blood.

Animals. The mice were Swiss albino animals from the Ness Ziona breeding colony, and were used when they reached a weight of 18 to 22 g. They were maintained on a diet of mouse pellets and water ad lib. The rabbits were both albino and colored animals from several sources in Israel, and were employed at different ages as indicated in the text. They were maintained on a diet of pellets, mixed greens and water. The guinea pigs were Hartley strain outbred animals from the Ness Ziona colony. They were also maintained on a diet of pellets, mixed greens and water. Both male and female animals were employed.

Studies on mice. Rabbits were immunized against *C. neoformans* by means of eight i.v. injections of 10^8 *C. neoformans* cells at intervals of three to four days. The first four injections consisted of heat-killed (80 C) cells; the last four of living cells. The rabbits were bled to obtain serum 10 days after the final inoculation. The agglutination titers of serum samples were determined by Evans' method (21).

The ring response was elicited in three- to eight-week-old male or female mice by the i.p. injection of 10^7 *C. neoformans* cells. The infecting culture was mixed in a ratio of 10 : 1 with IRS having a 1 : 300 agglutination titer. A total of 0.5 ml was injected.

Control animals received organisms exposed to normal rabbit serum, organisms treated with IRS which had been absorbed with the homologous strain or organisms not treated with serum. Groups of 10 to 20 mice were employed in the comparisons. The animals were killed at intervals after infection, and Giemsa-stained smears were made of the peritoneal exudate. Concurrently, a sample of the omentum was removed, stretched on a glass slide, immersed in methanol and stained by the Giemsa method.

In studies with radiolabeled cells, 3 μc of tritiated thymidine were administered i.p. to mice 24 hrs after the injection of 0.5 ml of mineral oil. Twenty-four hours later, serum-treated C. neoformans was injected by the same route. The omental spreads were fixed in methanol and autoradiographed for one to two weeks with Kodak AR 10 stripping film. The radiograms were then developed and stained as previously described (22).

For studies in tissue culture, monocytes were harvested from the peritoneal fluid of normal mice. 2.5 $\times$ 10^5 cells were suspended in Leighton tubes in a modified Chang (23) medium containing mouse embryo extract. After the cells had adhered to the glass, a suspension of 10^4 C. neoformans cells, pretreated with rabbit antiserum (final titer 1:32), was introduced into the tubes.

Studies in rabbits and guinea pigs. Phagocytic cells were derived from rabbits and guinea pigs by the i.p. injection of saline (50 and 20 ml, respectively); PMN cells were harvested 18 hr, and monocytes two to five days, after injection. For harvesting of cells, the abdominal cavity of an animal was opened and a large volume of Tyrode's solution instilled and later aspirated into a separatory funnel. After centrifugation, the phagocytic cells were counted and dispersed into Leighton tubes, in a maintenance medium composed of Tyrode's solution and 40% serum. For *in vitro* work, 0.5 $\times$ 10^6 PMN cells or 0.25 $\times$ 10^6 monocytes were mixed with 10^3 to 10^4 cryptococci. This ratio permitted the formation of multilayered rings around single yeast cells.

Viability studies on C. neoformans injected i.p. were conducted as follows: 3 $\times$ 10^7 or 3 $\times$ 10^6 yeast cells were injected into rabbits and guinea pigs, respectively. At various intervals the animals were opened and small pieces of the omentum (2 $\times$ 2 cm) were ground in sand and plated on Sabouraud's agar.

The following procedure was developed in order to determine the fate of cryptococci surrounded by leukocyte rings: cover glasses containing rings formed *in vitro* were placed on 60 mm plastic Petri dishes containing Sabouraud's agar, with the cells facing the medium. The rings could be observed easily at low magnification, and they were individually marked by means of a grid system engraved on the back of the Petri dishes. Twenty-four hours later the rings were examined. Dead cryptococci could easily be recognized, while viable cryptococci developed into microcolonies. Due to the anaerobic conditions prevailing under the cover glass, the development of the yeast cells was considerably slowed down, thus preventing the growth of one colony over the other. The same method was also applicable for rings formed *in vivo*. In these experiments, omentum was cut and spread on 22 × 40 mm cover glasses, which were then placed in the Petri dishes.

Staining of RNA was performed according to Kurnick (24) or Armstrong (25). For histochemical work, cover slips were employed either without fixation, or following 5 min fixation in 2% glutaraldehyde. Acid phosphatase activity was demonstrated by the procedure of Burstone (26) or by a modification of the Gomori method (27). Nonspecific esterase was demonstrated according to the method of Rozenszain et al. (28). For the reduction of tetrazolium salts, the procedure described in Pearse's "Histochemistry" was employed (29). Fixation and embedding for electron microscopy were performed according to the method of Edwards et al. (30).

RESULTS

Role of serum factors in ring formation. A) Immune serum in the mouse system: Mouse monocytes do not phagocytize or form rings around *C. neoformans* unless immune serum is added. M. Heidelberger has suggested (personal communication) that immune serum is necessary because of the slippery nature of the polysaccharide capsule. The serum component which is absorbed to the capsule presumably enables the pseudopodia of the phagocytes to adhere to its surface. This possibility was tested under both *in vitro* and *in vivo* conditions (20, 31).

The *in vitro* studies revealed the following: 1) Mouse peritoneal monocytes did not interact with small or large cryptococci without the addition of IRS. 2) In the presence of IRS two processes occurred concurrently: monocytes adhered to the cryptococci; and the cryptococci adhered to each other and agglutinated. Eventually, mixed aggregates of monocytes and yeast cells were obtained. 3) The best method for obtaining rings *in vitro* was to opsonize the cryptococci with IRS, to remove excess serum by centrifugation, and to add the treated cryptococci to a culture of monocytes. Rings were formed within 1 to 2 hr and persisted for several days, and no mixed aggregates were formed. 4) Opsonization of cryptococci with IRS with a low (1:5) agglutination titer was sufficient for ring formation. However, the structures thus obtained were very unstable. A mere tilting of the tubes sufficed to expel the enclosed cryptococci from the rings. 5) On the other hand, opsonization with IRS with a higher titer (1:300) resulted in the formation of three-dimensional structures; in other words, in this case the monocytes settled on top of the yeast cells as well as around them. (Due to the large size of the parasite, the distinction between two-dimensional rings and three-dimensional structures is unmistakable.)

The *in vivo* experiments gave essentially the same results as the *in vitro* study. Here again, only high titer serum caused the formation of three-dimensional structures, and also agglutinated cryptococci into large masses.

In summary, the results of these experiments are in agreement with the suggestion that the necessity for opsonization is connected with the slippery nature of the capsule. A small amount of IRS is sufficient for ring formation, but not sufficient to hold the cryptococci firmly. Moderate concentrations of IRS are adequate for obtaining stable but only two-dimensional rings; three-dimensional rings are formed only with high-titer serum.

B) Nonspecific opsonins in rabbit, guinea pig and human serum: In contrast to the observations made on mice, the addition of immune serum was not required for ring formation in rabbits and guinea pigs, either *in vitro* or *in vivo*. In both species two-dimensional rings were obtained, indicating that the opsonins in the nonimmunized rabbit and guinea pig are sufficient for obtaining stable rings but not sufficient for enclosing the parasite from all sides. The serum of all tested animals was checked prior to the experiments for its agglutinating capacity and for its ability to promote ring formation in mice. Both tests were invariably negative.

Characterization of the rabbit serum opsonin was attempted by fractionation experiments. Only preliminary data are so far available, however, because of the extreme lability of this factor (unpublished results). The opsonin in normal rabbit serum was inactivated by heating to 56 C for 30 min, and was lost as a result of storage at –20 C for several months and upon dialysis against saline in the cold. Our working hypothesis based on these preliminary data is that this opsonin may be identical with the nonspecific opsonin described by Hirsch (32), which is a pseudo-β globulin.

Under all the conditions in which the serum promoted formation of rings, phagocytosis was also observed, and vice-versa. It therefore seems plausible that the same factor enables the pseudopodia either to engulf the smaller cryptococci or to attach themselves to the surface of the larger yeast cells.

Human serum was similar to rabbit and guinea pig serum, both in its ability to promote the formation of rings and phagocytosis, and in the lability of its opsonin. Since patients suffering from leukemia are often prone to fungal infections, the opsonizing ability of the serum of eight leukemic patients was compared to that of five normal control subjects. However, no significant differences were found within this small sample.

The cellular response of rabbits and guinea pigs to the i.p. inoculation of C. neoformans. The sequence of cellular events in response to the i.p. injection of *C. neoformans* was studied in the rabbit and the guinea pig

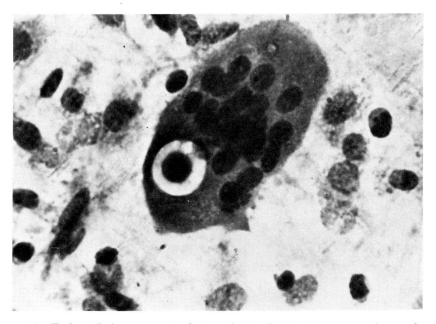

FIG. 2. Fusion of ring monocytes into a giant cell. Omentum preparation made three days after injection of *C. neoformans* into a rabbit. Giemsa stain. × 420. Reproduced with permission from SHAHAR A et al. *Isr J Med Sci* 5: 1164, 1969.

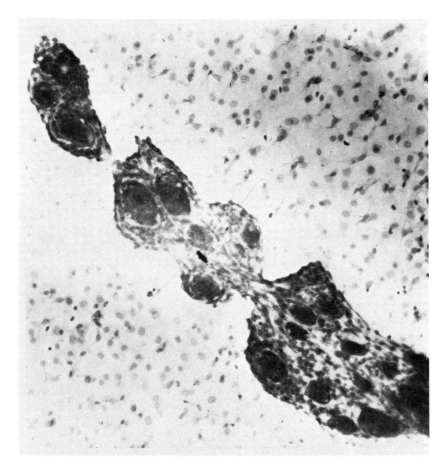

FIG. 3. Aggregation of small granulomata into larger ones. Spread of omentum prepared six days after injection of the yeast. Giemsa stain. × 250. Reproduced with permission from SHAHAR A et al. *Isr J Med Sci* **5**: 1164, 1969.

rather than in the mouse (31). Our choice was based on the assumption that in the mouse, which requires IRS for ring formation, mixed cellular-humoral reactions would occur. The cellular reactions were studied on stretch preparations of omentum.

In both species of animal, the cellular reaction following i.p. injection of the yeast began within a few hours, with migration of PMN cells. *In vitro* studies indicated that PMN cells were chemotactically attracted to the yeast cells. Both *in vitro* and *in vivo*, rings were initially formed by

PMN cells, but within 12 to 48 hr monocytes replaced the PMN cells. The mechanism of this replacement is not clear. Cellular cannibalism is thought to be involved, since monocytes containing remnants of PMN cells were occasionally seen. Tissue culture studies also revealed that the free monocytes move towards the PMN rings and, on arrival, push the latter away.

After the formation of monocyte rings, the cellular response follows completely different patterns in the two species. In the guinea pig, a few concentric rings of monocytes are formed within several days, after which there is no additional change with time (up to three weeks). In contrast, the monocytes often fuse into giant cells in the rabbit (Fig. 2) and granulomata are formed which tend to grow with time. Aggregation of these granulomata sometimes takes place, with the formation of collagen fibers; and the outgrowth of capillaries as bands connecting neighbouring foci (Fig. 3). However, fusion of ring monocytes was never seen in tissue culture, nor was a tendency to aggregation of rings observed under such experimental conditions as prolonged cultivation, addition of IRS and increase in the concentration of rings. In guinea pigs (and mice) fusion was observed neither *in vivo* nor *in vitro*.

To summarize: the first stages of the cellular response were more or less as expected and included the formation of PMN rings and their replacement by monocyte rings. However, with time, marked differences were observed between the rabbit and the guinea-pig and between *in vivo* and *in vitro* conditions in the rabbit. The factors which participate in the chronic reaction observed in the rabbit are not yet fully understood.

Fate of C. neoformans in the rabbit and the guinea pig. A) *In vivo* studies: Our earlier experiments (31) showed that cryptococci which are injected i.p. into rabbits are generally destroyed within 18 to 24 hr (Table 1). In the guinea pig, the cryptococci survived longer and an increased rate of killing of ring-enclosed cryptococci was noted between the second and the third days (Table 2).

These observations are in accord with the assumption (see Introduction) that the rabbit's resistance to *C. neoformans* is related to its high body temperature (39.5 C, as compared with the guinea-pig's temperature of 37 C). The effect of temperature in destroying the parasite therefore required clarification. Since normal serum from different species contains cryptococcidal substances (17, 18), the effect of both temperature and serum were studied in combination.

B) Effect of temperature at various serum concentrations on the viabil-

TABLE 1. *Viability of* C. neoformans *following i.p. injection into rabbits*

Age of rabbit	Hr afer injection	No. of cryptococci injected	No. of cryptococcus colonies[a]
4 to 6 months	2	3 × 10⁷	1,000
,,	2	,,	3,000
,,	2	,,	4,000
,,	4	,,	1,600
,,	4	,,	600
,,	6	,,	200
,,	8	1 × 10⁸	230
,,	8	,,	60
,,	18	,,	10
,,	,,	,,	0
,,	,,	3 × 10⁷	50
,,	,,	,,	900
,,	,,	1 × 10⁸	1,000
,,	,,	,,	75
7 days	,,	1 × 10⁷	100
,,	,,	,,	30
,,	,,	,,	20
4 to 6 months	24	1 × 10⁸	0
,,	,,	,,	0

[a] Plating was on Sabouraud agar from serial dilutions of sand-ground pieces of omentum measuring about 6 cm². The numbers are the average counts of triplicate samples from each rabbit.

ity of *C. neoformans*: The yeast grows much more slowly at 37 C than at 28 C in Sabouraud's medium, and is gradually inactivated at 39.5 C (Table 3). In the presence of serum, the yeast fails to grow even at 28 C, and is already inactivated at 37 C.

Most of the yeast cells are inactivated by rabbit serum *in vitro* at about the same time that they are destroyed under *in vivo* conditions. It is therefore not necessarily the ring structure itself which is operative in destroying the parasite in the rabbit, and the cryptococcidal activity of the rings could indeed be demonstrated only under special *in vitro* conditions.

No difference was found between the inhibitory power of serum from the nonsusceptible rabbit or guinea pig and from the mouse which is

TABLE 2. *Destruction of ring-encircled cryptococci in the peritoneum of guinea pigs*

Hr after injection	No. of cryptococci injected	No. of dead (encircled) cryptococci/total no. of rings	% of destruction
24	10^7	0/20	0
24	10^7	3/8	30
20	10^7	7/40	17
24	2×10^6	7/56	12
24	2×10^6	47/260	18
48	3×10^6	40/70	55
48	10^7	51/116	43
48	10^7	16/44	36
48	10^6	143/178	80
48	3×10^6	31/36	86
48	3×10^6	84/107	80
48	3×10^6	391/560	70
72	3×10^6	85/85	100

Pieces of omentum were spread on cover slips which were then inverted on Petri dishes containing Sabouraud's agar. Rings were individually marked. After 24 hr of incubation the plates were scored.

TABLE 3. *Colony counts of* C. neoformans *at various serum concentrations and temperatures as a function of time*

Incubation time (hr)	Sabouraud[a]			Sabouraud containing 25% serum[a]			Serum (100%)[a]		
	28C	37C	39.5C	28C	37C	39.5C	28C	37C	39.5C
0	220	220	220	190	190	190	230	230	230
3	200	200	205	180	185	195	180	150	185
9	225	190	220	205	190	180	205	160	180
24	400×10^2	100×10^2	85	225	135	55	250	50	30
48	100×10^3	600×10^2	5	205	90	60	240	5	5
72	220×10^4	260×10^3	10	370	100	20	270	5	0

[a] Medium.

susceptible to cryptococcus. Preliminary, unpublished experiments have shown that whereas the inhibitory properties of serum upon *Candida albicans* may be largely ascribed to transferrin (33), the situation is different with respect to *C. neoformans*. In the case of *C. albicans*, the

TABLE 4. *Effect of transferrin on the growth of* C. albicans *and* C. neoformans

Medium	No. of cells of C. albicans at			No. of cells of C. neoformans at		
	0 hr	24 hr	48 hr	0 hr	24 hr	48 hr
Serum alone	1.6×10^3	4.5×10^4	6.8×10^5	1.1×10^3	5.2×10^2	3×10^2
Serum + $(NH_4)_2 \cdot Fe(SO_4)_2$	1.6×10^3	8×10^4	3.4×10^7	1.1×10^3	4.5×10^2	2×10^2
Serum + transferrin	1.6×10^3	4.4×10^4	7.2×10^5	1.1×10^3	5.5×10^2	4.5×10^2
Serum + transferrin + 5 μg Fe^{++}	1.6×10^3	1×10^5	2.4×10^7	1.1×10^3	7×10^2	3.5×10^2
Serum + transferrin + 1 μg Fe^{++}	1.6×10^3	1.5×10^5	8×10^6	1.1×10^3	6.5×10^2	2.5×10^2

All media also contained glucose and ascorbic acid.
Details of experimental procedure are according to Caroline et al. (33).

addition of transferrin increased the serum's inhibitory power, while the addition of iron abolished it. Neither of these reactions took place with *C. neoformans* (Table 4). The absolute requirement of iron by the two yeasts is markedly different, and *C. neoformans* may grow for many generations in a medium containing only 0.1 μg of FeCl$_2$/ml, a concentration which does not permit the multiplication of *C. albicans*. Transferrin is therefore not the main serum factor inhibitory for *C. neoformans* but it is not impossible that it may act in conjunction with other factors.

Since serum destroys cryptococci at 37 C, it seemed puzzling that the parasite nevertheless multiplied in the mouse. It was noted, however, that lysates prepared by freezing and thawing red cells could abolish the serum inhibition (Table 5). Thus, in spite of the inhibitory power of serum, under certain conditions the parasite can develop in the tissue of the host.

Fate of C. neoformans *surrounded by leukocyte rings* in vitro. Serum at high temperature inactivates *C. neoformans in vitro* in about the same period of time required for the yeast to be destroyed *in vivo*. In order to show that the formation of leukocyte rings serves as a defense mechanism, conditions had to be found under which the serum itself

TABLE 5. Colony counts of C. neoformans on various media

Incubation time (hr)	Sabouraud[a]		Rabbit serum (100%)[a]		Whole rabbit blood[a]		Lysate of rabbit blood cells[a]	
	28C	37C	28C	37C	28C	37C	28C	37C
0	325	325	325	325	325	325	325	325
18	710×10^2	330×10^2	320	170	610×10	415	515×10	410×10
24	410×10^3	635×10^2	380	285	710×10	760	205×10^2	390×10
48	170×10^4	315×10^3	310	65	320×10^2	470×10	570×10^2	270×10^2
72	305×10^4	545×10^3	100	5	470×10^2	700×10	375×10^3	500×10^2

[a] Growth medium.

TABLE 6. *Destruction of* C. neoformans *by rabbit and guinea pig PMN rings under in* vitro *conditions*

| | Hours of exposure of cryptococci to action of ring cells | | | | | |
| | 2 | | 4 | | 6 | |
Animal	No. of dead (encircled) cryptococci/ total no. of rings	% destruction observed in rings	No. of deal (encircled) cryptococci/ total no. of rings	% destruction observed in rings	No. of dead (encircled) cryptococci/ total no. of rings	% destruction observed in rings
Rabbit	0/80	0	1/31	3	12/112	11
Rabbit	0/55	0	0/35	0	3/31	9
Rabbit	0/73	0	2/69	3	1/49	2
Rabbit	0/109	0	6/138	4	10/260	4
Guinea pig	0/120	0	0/40	0	0/39	0
Guinea pig	0/150	0	0/25	0	0/42	0

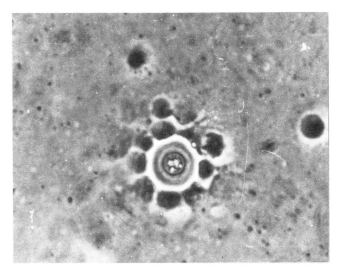

FIG. 4. Remnants of a dead, ring-encircled *C. neoformans* cell from an *in vitro* cover glass preparation. × 500. For technical details see Materials and Methods.

is not fungicidal. Under conditions in which the phagocytes were maintained *in vitro* in the presence of serum, the viability of the yeast cells was not diminished even after several days of incubation. The fate of cryptococci surrounded by rings was, therefore, studied in this system.

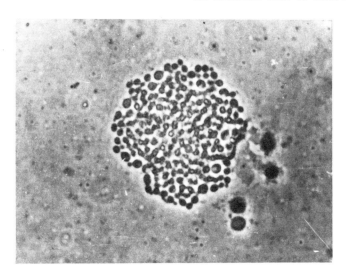

FIG. 5.   Microcolony of *C. neoformans* cells which developed from a viable, ring-encircled yeast cell from an *in vitro* cover glass preparation. × 500. For technical details see Materials and Methods.

In studies on the effect of PMN cells on encircled yeast cells *in vitro,* the experiments were of relatively short duration (8 hr exposure of the cryptococci to the action of ring cells). PMN cells are short-lived and we wished to avoid working with disintegrating phagocytes. Rabbit and guinea pig PMN phagocytes formed rings within 1 to 2 hr after introduction into tubes. Most of the cryptococci were surrounded by several (three to five) rows of cells and most of the encircled cells remained viable (Table 6) as in the *in vivo* study.

In contrast, Table 7 shows that encircling monocytes are able to destroy the surrounded yeast cells (Fig. 4 and 5). The process of destruction is slow; not more than 3 to 5% of the yeast cells lose their viability within 3 to 5 hr after becoming enclosed in rings, and one to two days' exposure were required for 50% killing. Cryptococci free of monocytes, which could be identified at this stage, were all viable. The encircling cells remained viable and active, as evidenced by their ability to ingest bacteria even at the stage when many cryptococci had already been destroyed.

In a few experiments in which monocytes were maintained in culture for two to three days prior to the addition of yeast cells, there was increased destruction of the latter. Likewise, monocytes harvested five

TABLE 7. *Destruction of* C. neoformans *by rabbit monocytic rings* in vitro. *Number of dead cryptococci/number of rings*

Identification no. of rabbit	No. of hr during which cryptococci were exposed to action of rings cells			
	3	24	48	72
1	0/95 (0)[a]	21/96 (22)	—	
2	0/150 (0)	17/182 (9.5)	—	
3	18/540 (3)	58/604 (10)	203/758 (27)	
3[b]	0/110 (0)	76/373 (20)	—	69/93 (74)
3[c]	5/108 (4)	48/117 (41)	104/163 (64)	
4	8/166 (5)	29/97 (30)	104/188 (55)	135/155 (87)
4[b]	0/120 (0)	29/34 (85)	80/104 (77)	
4[c]	0/115 (0)	44/62 (70)	—	
5	4/100 (4)	60/200 (30)	—	
6	0/155 (0)	2/40 (5)	115/359 (32)	
7	14/615 (2)	51/425 (12)	133/291 (46)	
8	8/652 (1)	35/302 (11)	147/336 (44)	
9	0/180 (0)	18/130 (14)	—	
10	0/95 (0)	20/65 (31)	—	
11[c]	0/80 (0)	17/25 (68)	—	

[a] Numbers in parentheses are percentages.
[b] Cryptococci were added to monocytes explanted 24 hr earlier.
[c] Cryptococci were added to monocytes explanted 48 hr earlier.

days after the i.p. injection of the saline stimulant were more active in destroying the yeast than those harvested after only two days. Previous exposure of rabbits to C. *neoformans* did not accelerate the destruction of yeast cells either *in vitro* or *in vivo*.

Since guinea-pig monocytes did not maintain themselves well in culture, these experiments were performed only with rabbit monocytes.

The secretion of enzymes by encircling cells. When large parasites are encapsulated in the body of insects, asphyxia is considered to be the most common mode of parasite destruction (34). Such encapsulation in insects is characterized by the presence of many layers of hematocytes around the parasites.

It was previously emphasized that the ring of phagocytic cells is two-dimensional in normal, nonimmunized animals, and thus the parasite may obtain oxygen and metabolites through its free upper part. Since asphyxia is accordingly ruled out, it was assumed that phagocytic cell secretions

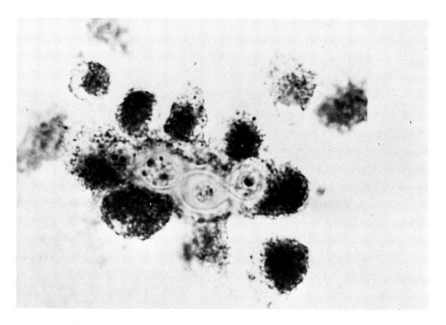

FIG. 6. Acid phosphatase release by ring monocytes into the surrounded chain of yeast cells. Note the granular appearance of the reaction product and the dense precipitate in the enclosed cryptococci. *In vitro* cover slip preparation. Staining performed according to Burstone's technique (26). × 1,000.

have cryptococcidal properties in our model. Since monocytes encircling yeasts are much more basophilic than free monocytes, increased protein synthesis in the former was suspected. Indeed, staining with methyl green-pyronin (24, 25) showed that encircling monocytes possess a higher RNA content than free monocytes.

One possible explanation of the intense staining of encircling cells might be that they are preparing for division, and the outer rings in the multilayered structures would thus originate from division of cells in the inner layers. If this were indeed so, labeling of some cells of the inner rings with tritiated thymidine should result in a radially-arranged labeling of the multilayered ring structure. If, on the other hand, the outer rings of encircling monocytes are formed by the migration of monocytes and not by their division, the labeling should be random. Our results (20) suggest that the cells indeed migrate rather than divide.

We next attempted to establish whether the encircling cells secrete proteins. For this purpose enzymes which can be demonstrated histochem-

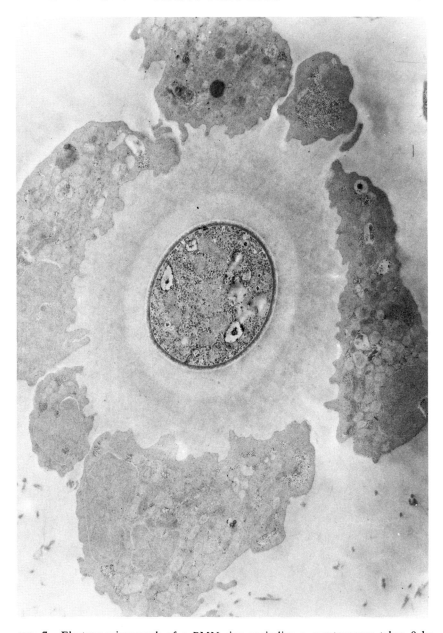

FIG. 7. Electron micrograph of a PMN ring encircling a cryptococcus taken 8 hr after i.p. injection into a rabbit. The yeast cell's organelles are still visible. Note penetration of pseudopodia into the capsule. Fixation, embedding and preparation for electron microscopy according to Edwards et al. (30). × 6,700.

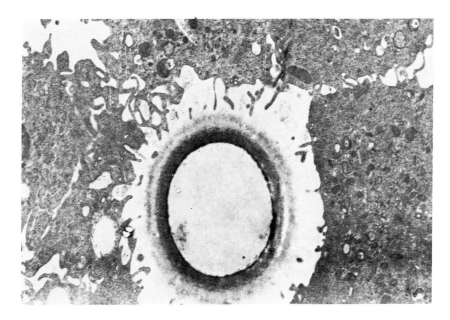

FIG. 8.   Electron micrograph of a monocyte ring encircling a cryptococcus taken three days after i.p. injection into a rabbit. All organelles have disappeared. Note deep penetration of pseudopodia into the capsule. Fixation, embedding and preparation for electron microscopy according to Edwards et al. (30). × 6,700.

ically were chosen. These experiments were conducted with both PMN cells and monocytes of rabbit and guinea-pig, *in vitro* and also *in vivo*. The cryptococci were preheated to 90 C, in order to abolish their own enzymatic activity.

Several enzymes were found to accumulate in the encircling phagocytes at sites near the cryptococci. The presence of these enzymes was also demonstrated within the encircled cryptococci, whereas neighbouring free cryptococci showed no enzymatic activity or only traces of activity (35) (Fig. 6). The phagocytes were thought to secrete these enzymes in the vicinity of the parasite. The enzymes which were secreted by both PMN cells and monocytes *in vitro* and *in vivo*, were all hydrolytic: β-glycerophosphatase (27), naphthol As-Bi phosphatase (26) and esterase (28).

Electron micrographs taken three days after the injection of cryptococci into rabbits revealed the complete disappearance of organelles from the engulfed cryptococcus (Fig. 7 and 8). It is possible that the secreted enzymes participated in the digestion of the killed yeast cells. The same

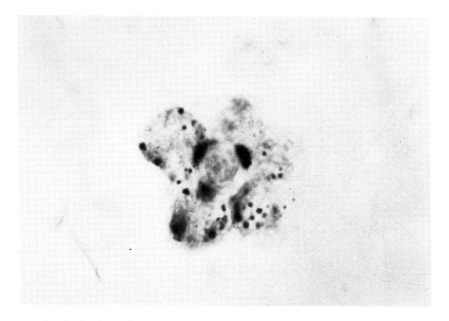

FIG. 9. Reduction of nitroblue tetrazolium chloride by monocytes encircling a cryptococcus. *In vitro* cover slip preparation. Note an intense augmentation of tetrazolium reduction at the region of contact of three of the monocytes with the yeast cell. For technical details see Pearse's "Histochemistry" (29). × 1,000.

enzymes were also demonstrated within cryptococci phagocytized by monocytes. (PMN cells can hardly ingest even the small cryptococci.) Since PMN cells are end cells and short-lived, enzyme release could have been the result of a "suicidal" behavior (36). The viability of the encircling PMN cells was demonstrated, since they are capable of phagocytizing and destroying bacteria such as *Staphylococcus albus, Escherichia coli* and *Bacillus subtilis*. In other words, the encircling cells, which released hydrolytic enzymes towards the enclosed cryptococci, remained viable and functional.

Numerous observations on encircling cells under phase contrast illumination at 37 C failed to demonstrate extrusion of lysosomes from the cells. Marked activity of the pseudopodia at the surface of the yeast capsule could, however, be seen. Ultrastructural studies indeed showed that such pseudopodia penetrate into the yeast capsule (Fig. 7, 8). Moreover, histochemical studies of the encircling cells revealed increased oxidative activity. This was shown by a dramatic increase in the reducton of nitroblue tetrazolium salt (29) at the site of contact between the pseudopodia and the yeast (Fig. 9).

Our discussion is centered on three problems: a) the role of opsonin in the development of cellular rings which are formed around cryptococci; b) the analogy between classical phagocytosis and the ring reaction; and c) the nature of the host-parasite relationship in cryptococcosis.

C. neoformans was employed as a model in order to study vertebrate host response to large-sized parasites. The cellular aspects of the host response were studied mainly on the omentum, permitting preservation of the architecture of the complex cellular reactions which follow the injection of cryptococci without the introduction of artifacts. The model is suitable for cytochemical studies and for electron microscopy, although the embedding problems common with yeasts are encountered. Furthermore, the existence of both susceptible and resistant hosts permits comparative studies.

Our results justify the assumption that opsonization of the yeast is required for mechanical reasons, namely, to provide the pseudopodia of the phagocyte with a hold on the slippery yeast capsule.

Opsonins are generally thought to aid in the discrimination between "self" and "nonself." In the mouse, the phagocytic cells did not recognize the cryptococci as "foreign"; they never attempted to phagocytize them, but completely ignored them. It would seem that much less opsonin is needed for recognition than for the formation of stable rings. Rowley has shown that as few as eight molecules of IgM are needed for the recognition of *Salmonella typhimurium* by mouse macrophages (37).

The importance of mechanical aspects in phagocytosis was shown long ago in the phenomenon of surface phagocytosis (38) in a model in which another slippery capsule was involved, that of the pneumococcus. When phagocytes and bacteria are mixed in test tubes, no phagocytosis occurs without the presence of immune serum. In the presence of a solid surface (such as cellular fibers) the phagocytes can push the bacteria against the surface and ingest them even in the absence of antibody.

Our experiments with IRS, both *in vitro* and *in vivo,* showed that the high-titer serum has a dual effect, one to the host's advantage and the other to its disadvantage. On the one hand, the parasite becomes completely surrounded by phagocytes. On the other hand, the same serum agglutinates the cryptococci into very large masses which cannot be effectively handled by the host's cells. This might perhaps explain the results of Gadebusch's experiments, also confirmed by us, that the injection of immune serum into mice infected with *C. neoformans* prolonged the animals' lives without curing them (15).

On the whole, we observed a good correlation between the agglutinating titer of the IRS and its opsonizing capacity. However, in one rabbit a serum of very low titer proved to be very effective as an opsonin. This suggests the possibility that the two activities, opsonization and agglutination, are distinct. Opsonizing serum devoid of agglutinating properties would be presumed to have better therapeutic value, since it would achieve a cellular reaction against the parasite without, at the same time, causing large clumps of the latter to form. An interesting possibility suggested to us by M. Shilo was to use a monovalent antibody which would presumably opsonize the yeasts without agglutinating them.

The formation of rings of phagocytes surrounding large objects was considered by us to be analogous to the phagocytosis of small objects. The process of phagocytosis, though continuous, is generally divided into sequential stages. Even though somewhat arbitrary, these stages are very convenient in distinguishing the mechanisms involved in phagocytosis and they also serve in comparing phagocytosis with the ring phenomenon.

1) Chemotaxis (although not yet clearly demonstrated under *in vivo* conditions) is believed to be the first step in phagocytosis, the phagocytes migrating from a distance towards a stimulant. Our tissue culture studies indeed showed that those PMN cells which eventually form rings do not reach the cryptococci at random but actively migrate towards them.

2) The presence of PMN cells and their products generally induces the migration of monocytes. These arrive after several hours, and phagocytize the PMN cells. In the ring system, encircling PMN cells are replaced after 12 to 18 hr by encircling monocytes and the monocytes phagocytize some of the PMN cells.

3) Opsonization is necessary for the phagocytes to distinguish self from nonself, and also to tackle slippery organisms. Since in our model the size of the cryptococci could be controlled at will, the same species of parasite was used for comparative studies, with size as a variable. It was indeed found that the same serum or serum fraction either promoted both phagocytosis and ring formation or neither of these activities. In

the mouse, neither phagocytosis nor ring formation occurred, but with the addition of immune serum both phenomena were observed.

4) The engulfment of particles by phagocytes is preceded by the attachment of the phagocytes' pseudopodia to the particles. By definition, in the ring phenomenon only pseudopodial attachment occurs, and engulfment by individual cells does not take place. Attachment is, nonetheless, quite stable when sufficient opsonin is present. The cryptococci are held firmly by the encircling cells and are not dislodged from the center of the ring either by tilting or by centrifugation of the tubes. The pseudopodia actually penetrate deeply into the capsule.

5) After phagocytosis is achieved, lysosomes fuse with phagosomes and lysosomal enzymes are released into the common vacuole and participate in the breakdown of the engulfed particle. In the rings, too, lysosomal enzymes are released in the direction of the parasite. Presumably, cryptococcidal substances are released in the same manner. The possibility that lysozyme is the substance responsible for destroying the cryptococci is being investigated. The hydrolytic enzymes released are thought to participate in the degradation of the yeast's organelles.

6) Phagocytosis is generally followed by an increase in oxygen uptake and in metabolic activity, and by a shift in the glycolytic pathway leading to H_2O_2 formation (39). Our attempts to demonstrate the formation of free H_2O_2 have not been successful (unpublished data). However, a very marked increase in the reduction of tetrazolium salt was noted in pseudopodia of monocytes in the region of contact with the cryptococcus. Whether this increase in oxidative metabolism is analogous to the metabolic changes following phagocytosis, or whether it represents increased pseudopodial activity near the parasite, is still an open question.

7) Finally, phagocytosis is the defense mechanism par excellence against small parasites. We have queried whether the ring reaction may be considered as an analogous defense mechanism against large parasites, resulting in the latter's destruction. Our own and others' experimental evidence shows that the host defense in cryptococcosis is quite complex. Serum factors, antibody, lysozyme, temperature and PMN cationic proteins may all be involved, and it is not possible at the moment to evaluate the relative contribution of each factor under *in vivo* conditions. On the other hand we have shown that under certain *in vitro* conditions the encircling cells are capable of destroying the yeast. This process requires a relatively long time. In freshly formed monocyte rings, only 3 to 5% of the encircled cryptococci were destroyed; and a further 24 to 48 hr

exposure of the cryptococci to the action of the encircling monocytes was required for 50% killing. Our *in vitro* experiments with PMN cells were of short duration (8 hr) to avoid working with disintegrating cells, and under these conditions destruction of cryptococci was minimal. It is quite likely that when the PMN cells are replaced by monocytes *in vivo,* the disintegration of the former may contribute to the destruction of cryptococci. In the guinea pig, most of the destruction of the cryptococcus takes place at the stage when the yeast is encircled by monocytes, and the latter may perhaps be more important than the PMN cells in killing the parasite. A possible mechanism of destruction is the secretion of cryptococcidal substances from the phagocytes. Since the killing action of phagocytes is slow, one might have expected the yeast cells to bud and demolish the encircling rings before the ring cells could destroy them. However, the fungistatic activity of the serum inhibits the growth of the yeast, thus permitting the encircling cells to exert their fungicidal activity, which leads to the ultimate destruction of the parasite.

Cryptococci tend to be opportunists rather than true pathogens, and cryptococcosis is rather rare, even when potential hosts are exposed to the microorganism. A variety of factors which interfere with normal defense mechanisms have been implicated in predisposing the host to infection. *C. neoformans* has no known mechanisms of virulence, such as toxins or specific enzymes which actively damage the host, destroy its defense mechanisms or lyse its tissues with consequent liberation of metabolites for the parasite's growth. Thus, occasional large masses of cryptococci are observed without any apparent damage to the surrounding tissues.

The microorganism is nevertheless endowed with several properties which enable it to survive and even to proliferate in the host. These properties are probably connected with the presence of the capsule, which under *in vivo* conditions may grow to a size well beyond that of the phagocytic cells and fend off phagocytes mechanically. In addition, the capsular material may induce a state of "immune paralysis."

C. neoformans might possibly be regarded as representing an intermediate stage between a typical saprophyte and a typical pathogen, its adaptation to parasitic life being confined to the acquisition of defense mechanisms against the host, rather than to directly offensive ones. Even in a susceptible host, the progress of cryptococcosis is slow and it may take months before the host dies. The slow progress is not connected with slow proliferation of the yeast; whereas in other chronic infectious diseases, such as tuberculosis or leprosy, the parasite grows very sluggishly, *C. neoformans* grows quite rapidly, with a generation time of 2 to 3 hr. There is a considerable variety of tissue reactions by different hosts to cryptococcus. Tissue responses were relatively stable in individuals of the same species, but there was a considerable difference in the reactions of the three species studied, mouse, guinea pig and rabbit. For many of the tissue responses in man (no discernible reaction, accumulation of monocytes and formation of giant cells) there is a counterpart in one or more of the experimental animals.

We assume that the variety of tissue reactions observed may be connected with the opportunistic nature of the pathogen. Many factors, humoral as well as cellular, can confer resistance against the parasite. Cryptococcosis develops when one or more of these mechanisms weakens or fails. The pathological manifestations of the disease in a given case quite possibly reflect the operation of the mechanisms still available, which may vary from one case to the other. The pattern of host reaction and the course of a disease are likely to be more uniform and predictable when a true pathogen is involved than when an opportunist invades a previously weakened subject.

A careful comparison of the specific tissue reactions in man with the analogous reactions in experimental animals, preferably at the early stages, may perhaps tell us which of the protective mechanisms are (and which ones are not) operating in the human disease.

Frequently, no tissue reaction to cryptococcus can be seen in man. This is also the typical situation in the mouse, and it is associated in that animal with lack of opsonins. Whether the serum of human cryptococcosis patients lacks opsonins is not known. If opsonins should prove to be present in the human host, cells of the RES may possibly have been adversely affected by immunosuppressive treatment for a predisposing disease.

When a cellular response does occur in human cryptococcosis patients, the predominant cell is the histiocyte. In the human disease, histiocytes remain separate in some cases, whereas in others they fuse into giant cells. It is presumed that giant cells are particularly effective against the parasite since they completely enclose it. In the guinea pig, encircling histiocytes remain separate, whereas in the rabbit they also fuse into giant cells. However, under *in vitro* conditions rabbit monocytes were never observed to fuse even under a wide variety of experimental circumstances. Certain factors may be required specifically, for such fusion to occur.

Finally, it has been suggested before (12, 13) and corroborated in the present work that C. *neoformans* is susceptible to high temperatures (> 37 C). In the past, attempts to cure the disease by elevating the patients' body temperature were not very successful because elevated temperatures would have to be maintained for a prolonged period. Nevertheless, it remains tempting to exploit the susceptibility of the yeast to heat. Thus, for example, it might be possible to attain prolonged *local* elevation of temperature by infrared irradiation focused upon the lesion.

SUMMARY

This study deals with a host-parasite relationship involving a large-sized pathogen, *Cryptococcus neoformans*, which offers a particularly useful model for investigating the cellular responses of the host. The effects on the development of this yeast *in vitro* exerted by temperature, serum and nutritional factors, and the reactions of various animal species were studied. The pattern of response in all of the species studied was similar: The cryptococci, introduced into the peritoneum, were first surrounded by rings formed of polymorphonuclear cells, and these were later replaced by rings of monocytes. Under mild opsonization, the host cells merely surrounded the cryptococci but did not settle on them; the rings thus remained two-dimensional. With larger quantities of opsonizing antibody three-dimensional rings were formed, completely encapsulating the cryptococci. Ring monocytes were much more basophilic than free monocytes.

The ring response, which occurred naturally in guinea pigs and rabbits, required the addition of immune (rabbit) serum for elicitation in the mouse, since this animal does not produce the specific opsonins. The need for opsonization apparently stems from the slippery nature of the yeast's capsule; the pseudopodia of phagocytes cannot attach themselves to the parasite without opsonin.

The increased basophilia of the ring monocytes is related to increased protein synthesis. One of the mechanisms involved in destroying the ring-enclosed cryptococci is attributed to this increased protein synthesis; release of enzymes from the phagocytes into the parasite is demonstrable histochemically. The phagocytes which release enzymes are intact, functioning cells.

In the guinea-pig and the mouse, little additional change takes place after the rings are formed. In the rabbit, however, the ring monocytes often fuse into giant cells within three to four days, and these in turn, aggregate into large granulomata.

Cryptococci are destroyed much more rapidly in the rabbit than in the guinea-pig. Serum factors and temperature contribute largely to the rabbit's defense against the yeast. Under suitable *in vitro* conditions, ring monocytes are capable of destroying surrounded cryptococci, and similar monocytes may participate in the eventual destruction of the yeast in the guinea pig.

An analogy is drawn between phagocytosis as a defense mechanism against small organisms and the ring reaction as a response against larger ones.

The authors gratefully acknowledge the collaboration, at different stages of this work, of A. Beemer, J.J. Bubis, M. Helman, M. Kalima, S. Schneerson-Porath, A. Shahar, L. Shalish and Y. Sobel. We are indebted to M. Wolman for helpful discussions and advice in the preparation of this manuscript.

Supported in part by the Eshkol Scholarship Fund and by Grant AI–04991 from the National Institutes of Health, U.S. Public Health Service.

REFERENCES

1. METCHNIKOFF E. "Life of Elie Metchnikoff." Boston, Houghton Mifflin Co, 1921, pp 116–117.
2. MEKBEL S and VON LICHTENBERG F. Granuloma formation in the laboratory mouse. 11. Reaction to *A. suis* eggs in the presensitized host. *J Infect Dis* 110: 253–257, 1962.
3. VON LICHTENBERG F. Host responses to eggs of *S. mansoni*. I. Granuloma formation in the unsensitized laboratory mouse. *Am J Pathol* 41: 711–731, 1962.
4. WARREN KS, DOMINGO EO and COWAN RBT. Granuloma formation around schistosome eggs as a manifestation of delayed hypersensitivity. *Am J Pathol* 51: 735–756, 1967.
5. DOMINGO EO and WARREN KS. Endogenous desensitization: Changing host granulomatous response to schistosome eggs at different stages of infection with *Schistosoma mansoni*. *Am J Pathol* 52: 369–377, 1968.
6. LITTMAN ML and TSUBURA E. Effect of degree of encapsulation upon virulence of *Cryptococcus neoformans*. *Proc Soc Exp Biol Med* 101: 773–777, 1959.
7. EMMONS CW. Prevalence of *Cryptococcus neoformans* in pigeon habitats. *Public Health Rep* 75: 362–364, 1960.
8. LEVINE HB. Immunogenicity of experimental vaccines in systemic mycoses, in: Dalldorf G (Ed), "Fungi and fungus diseases." Springfield, Ill, Charles C Thomas, 1962, pp 254–276.
9. ABRAHAMS I and GILLERAN TG. Studies on actively acquired resistance to experimental cryptococcis in mice. *J Immunol* 85: 629–635, 1961.

10. FELTON LD and OTTINGER B. Pneumococcus polysaccharide as a paralyzing agent on the mechanism of immunity in white mice. *J Bacteriol* **43**: 94, 1942.
11. CAMPBELL CC. Serology in respiratory mycoses. *Sabouraudia* **5**: 240–259, 1967.
12. LITTMAN ML and ZIMMERMAN LE. "Cryptococcosis." New York, Grune and Stratton, 1956.
13. BERGMAN F. Effect of temperature on intratesticular cryptococcal infection in rabbits. *Sabouraudia* **5**: 54–58, 1966.
14. BULMER GS and SANS MD. *Cryptococcus neoformans.* II. Inhibition of phagocytosis. *J Bacteriol* **95**, 5–8, 1968.
15. GADEBUSH HH. Passive immunization against *Cryptococcus neoformans. Proc Soc Exp Biol Med* **98**: 611–614, 1958.
16. GADEBUSH HH and JOHNSON AG. Natural host resistance to infection with *Cryptococcus neoformans.* IV. The effect of some cationic proteins on the experimental disease. *J Infect Dis* **116**: 551–565, 1966.
17. IGEL HJ and BOLANDE RP. Humoral defense mechanisms in cryptococcus: substances in normal human serum, saliva, and cerebrospinal fluid affecting the growth of *Cryptococcus neoformans. J Infect Dis* **116**: 75–83, 1966.
18. REISS F and SZILAGI G. The effect of mammalian and avian sera on the growth of *Cryptococcus neoformans. J Invest Dermatol* **48**: 264–267, 1967.
19. AL-DOORY J. A bibliography of cryptococcosis, *Mycopathol Mycol Appl* **45**: 1–60, 1971.
20. SCHNEERSON-PORAT S, SHAHAR A and ARONSON M. Formation of histiocyte rings in response to *Cryptococcus neoformans* infection. *J Reticuloendothel Soc* **2**: 249–255, 1965.
21. EVANS EE. The antigenic composition of *Cryptococcus neoformans. J Immunol* **64**: 423–430, 1950.
22. ARONSON M and ELBERG SS. Proliferation of rabbit peritoneal histiocytes as revealed by autoradiography with tritiated thymidine. *Proc Natl Acad Sci USA* **48**: 208–214, 1962.
23. CHANG YT. The mouse macrophage as host cell for *Mycobacterium leprae. Symposium on Research in Leprosy, sponsored by the Leonard Wood Memorial and the Johns Hopkins University, Washington, 1961.*
24. ARMSTRONG JA. Histochemical differentiation of nucleic acid by means of induced fluorescence. *Exp Cell Res* **11**: 640–643, 1956.
25. KURNICK NB. Pyronin Y in the methyl-green-pyronin histochemical stain. *Stain Technol* **30**: 213–230, 1955.
26. BURSTONE MS. The relationship between fixation and techniques for the histochemical localization of hydrolytic enzymes. *J Histochem Cytochem* **6**: 322–339, 1958.
27. BITENSKY L. The demonstration of lysosomes by the controlled temperature freezing sectioning method. *Q J Microsc Sci* **103**: 205, 1962.
28. ROZENSZAIN L, LEIBOVICH M, SHOHAM D and EPSTEIN J. The esterase activity in megaloblasts and normal haemopoietic cells. *Br J Exp Pathol* **14**: 605–610, 1968.
29. PEARSE AGE. "Histochemistry: theoretical and applied," 2nd edn. London, Churchill Ltd, p 910.
30. EDWARDS MR, GORDON MA, LAPA EW and GHIORSE WC. Micromorphology of *Cryptococcus neoformans J Bacteriol* **94**: 766–777, 1967.
31. SHAHAR A, KLETTER Y and ARONSON M. Granuloma formation in cryptococcosis. *Isr J Med Sci* **5**: 1164–1172, 1969.
32. JOHNSTON RR, KLEMPERER MR, ALPER CA and ROSEN FS. The enhancement of bacterial phagocytosis by serum. *J Exp Med* **129**: 1275–1290, 1969.
33. CAROLINE L, ROSNER F and KOZINN APJ. Elevated serum iron, low unbound transferrin and candidiasis in acute leukemia. *Blood* **34**: 441–451, 1969.
34. SALT G. The defense reactions of insects to metazoan parasites. *Parasitology* **53**: 527–642, 1963.

162 M. ARONSON AND J. KLETTER

35. KALINA M, KLETTER Y, SHAHAR A and ARONSON M. Acid phosphatase release from intact phagocytic cells surrounding a large-sized parasite. *Proc Soc Exp Biol Med* **136**: 407–410, 1971.
36. ROWLEY D. Phagocytosis and immunity. *Experientia* **22**: 1–64, 1966.
37. SPICER SS and HARDIN JH. Ultrastructure, cytochemistry and function of neutrophil leukocyte granules. A review. *Lab Invest* **20**: 488–497, 1969.
38. SUTER E. Interaction between phagocytes and pathogenic microorganisms. *Bacteriol Rev* **20**: 94–132, 1956.
39. KLEBANOFF SJ. Myeloperoxidase-halide-hydrogen peroxide antibacterial system. *J Bacteriol* **95**: 2131–2138, 1968.

NONSPECIFIC STIMULATION OF ANTIMICROBIAL AND ANTITUMOR RESISTANCE AND OF IMMUNOLOGICAL RESPONSIVENESS BY THE MER FRACTION OF TUBERCLE BACILLI*

DAVID W. WEISS and DIANE J. YASHPHE

Department of Immunology and Lautenberg Center for General and Tumor Immunology, Hebrew University–Hadassah Medical School, Jerusalem, Israel

INTRODUCTION

MER (Methanol Extraction Residue) is a moiety of virulent, attenuated and avirulent tubercle bacilli which is capable of markedly increasing the resistance of experimental animals to microbial pathogens and to neoplastic cells of syngeneic and autochthonous origin, and of profoundly modulating immunological responsiveness to unrelated antigens. The substance holds considerable interest as a reliable model illustrating the possibility of elevating resistance states by nonspecific means and of broadly altering immunological reactivity in experimentally and clinically desirable directions. It may itself have direct and applied medical significance, and it appears to be a useful tool in the study of the mechanisms of immunological reactivity, including the magnification of otherwise minimal or undetectable reactions.

The development of MER well illustrates the fact that interesting scientific information is often attained by unintended and very indirect pathways. Because there may be some didactic value in a description of

---

* Until 1968, most of the expriments with MER here described were carried out by the senior author and his associates in the several laboratories in the U.S. and England mentioned in the text. The several studies of other investigators are identified as such. Since 1968, all work referred to as performed by us and in our laboratories pertains to investigations undertaken jointly by both authors and their colleagues in Israel.

[163]

the sequence of error, unforeseen incident and chance meeting which led to the recognition of MER as a powerful modulator of immunity, the story of its finding and biologic characterization will be told as it actually occurred, chronologically and without varnishing the elements of chance.

DEVELOPMENT OF THE MER FRACTION

The observations which led to the development of MER were made in the course of investigations designed to answer a problem which seemed to have no bearing on nonspecific immunity, immunological modulation or neoplasia. This problem was: Can some protection against tuberculous infection be bestowed on experimental animals by nonliving vaccines consisting of intact tubercle bacilli and bacillary fractions? This was suggested as a research topic to the senior author when he entered the laboratories of Dr. René J. Dubos at the Rockefeller Institute for Medical Research in 1952.*

At a time when tuberculosis was still the leading cause of death in most parts of the world, including technologically civilized ones, this question was of great pertinency, especially in light of the considerable dissatisfaction in which living BCG, the then available antituberculosis vaccine, was held in places beyond the sphere of influence of French science (1–3). An answer also promised to be of significance to the basic question of the mode of action of acquired antituberculosis immunity, especially with regard to the long-standing conflict as to whether delayed hypersensitivity to tuberculoproteins constitutes a major mechanism of resistance (a problem still not entirely resolved) (4).

A large literature prior to 1952, including reports of many well-designed experiments, already provided persuasive evidence that certain nonliving mycobacterial preparations could induce acquired immunity to the same limited extent as living, attenuated ones. Work from Dr. Dubos' laboratory had also shown that tubercle bacilli fully inactivated by phenol retained

---

* I have always suspected that this problem fell to me at least partly because of an unusual reputation which I earned as a graduate student at Rutgers University: Three years of mouth-pipetting highly virulent tubercle bacilli almost continuously, in the course of a study on the mode of action of an antibiotic agent, failed to bring about even a modest conversion to tuberculin positivity, and the heroic resistance to tuberculous infection indicated by this failure augured well for my capacity to survive in a project involving heavy exposure to these pathogens. — DWW.

immunogenicity in mice (3, 5). As is so often the case even in the natural sciences, however, fact may find itself disarmed by fiction, or at least by dogma. Living BCG, representing the first widely accepted antituberculosis prophylactic, and hallowed as it was by the dedication of its discoverers and the glories of Gallic scientific endeavor, came to be taken by many as vindication of the quite erroneous but hoary dictum that living vaccines are inherently superior. The comment of Pearson and Gilliland in 1902 that "the whole study of immunization has led investigators to suspect a solution to tuberculosis immunity through the use of a living virus" (6) is representative, and the view was canonized by later workers in the field. Even discerning investigators who were conscious of the historic basis of the bias concluded that the hope for effective antituberculosis vaccines lay with living preparations. [For example, Long wrote in 1926 (7): "The success of Pasteur with attenuated anthrax and chicken cholera germs had prepared the way, the example of Jenner was a constant stimulus . . . It is significant that among the very first studies were experiments on the immunizing properties of living tubercle bacilli. Immunity following infection was an unescapable clinical fact in the case of other diseases, and . . . the more dangerous method of immunizing appeared to many early investigators more likely to be effective than the use of specific material made harmless by heat, chemicals or other reason," and concluded that the hope for effective antituberculosis vaccines lay with living agents.] The climate of opinion in the 1950s was well summarized by Gaisford (8) who noted that "one has come to think in terms of BCG (living) when talking of protective vaccination against tuberculosis." Although attacking this position was something in the nature of tilting against windmills in view of the experimental information actually available, the joust was an uphill one, and necessary if the remnants of an obscurantist vitalism were to be removed from the field of tuberculosis research.

Among the earlier reports of effective vaccination against tuberculosis with a mycobacterial fraction were those of Negrè and Boquet, who worked with a methanol-soluble extract, "antigène méthylique" (9). On Dr. Dubos' suggestion, experiments were initiated by the senior author in 1953 to reproduce the findings of these workers and extend them sufficiently to provide, once and for all, a convincing argument for the immunizing efficacy of a bacillary fraction.

In the course of the next three years, extensive immunization experiments were conducted in mice with methanol extracts of the avirulent human strain H37Ra and of the attenuated bovine variety BCG. Living bacteria were employed as positive controls, and whole phenol-killed organisms as a prototype of intact, but nonliving, bacillary vaccines. The whole killed bacteria were consistently found to be as effective as the living ones (10–12), but the results with the extracts were ambiguous. The first preparations made were equally effective (11, 12), but subsequent ones often proved only minimally capable of conferring protection, or not at all. It then occurred to us that the activity only occasionally displayed by the extract might perhaps be due to small quantities of the residue contaminating the material at times as a result of insufficient care in preparation. Exploratory tests indeed revealed that the residue of the methanol extraction was almost invariably as potent as living or intact killed BCG, with a suggestion of even slightly greater ability. [Later work with guinea pigs also pointed to a synergistic effect of small quantities of the extract administered together with subeffective quantities of the residue (13).]

It is not at all certain whether methanol extracts of BCG, H37Ra and virulent strains of tubercle bacilli do, as a rule, owe their protective activity largely to contamination with residual methanol-insoluble material. There have been reports by other workers of the capacity of methanol extracts of mycobacteria to heighten resistance and stimulate immunological reactivity in different systems (9, 14–16), and it may well be that the extracts themselves possess immunogenic powers, specific and nonspecific. It is also possible that a factor in the extract represents a specific antituberculosis protective antigen, and that the methanol extraction residue, MER, acts as a nonspecific stimulator of resistance. In any event, our attention was now focused on the residue rather than on the product of methanol extraction of tubercle bacilli, and the senior author has been unable to escape from involvement with MER during the ensuing 15 years. Rather like a mistress too attractive to discard altogether, but not compelling enough to wed, MER has remained an ongoing but secondary interest in our laboratories, until it recently presented itself one morning with a license for permanency, a subject for serious involvement after all.

Three years of work with mice at the Rockefeller Institute using living and phenolized tubercle bacilli, methanol extracts and MER made it obvious once more that the nonliving organisms and crude fractions can indeed afford a degree of limited protection against experimental tuberculosis similar to that elicited by viable preparations. These observations answered the question initially posed, and the senior author then turned to a new approach towards elucidation of the mechanisms of acquired immunity to tuberculosis. This was to take advantage of the findings then recently described by Medawar and his co-workers that animals could be rendered permanently unresponsive to foreign antigens by exposure to them early in life (17). In collaboration with the late A. Q. Wells, attempts were initiated in 1955 at the Sir William Dunn School of Pathology at Oxford University to render guinea pigs immunologically tolerant to tuberculoproteins by prenatal contact, and to study tuberculosis immunogenesis and pathogenesis in such animals when they had reached early adulthood. It was hoped thus to compare the host-parasite relationship between the guinea pig and the tubercle bacillus in normal animals with that in animals specifically incapable of developing antibodies or delayed hypersensitivity to at least some of the proteins of the pathogen. The first series of experiments indeed indicated that guinea pigs injected *in utero* with the tubercle bacillus protein preparations known as OT (Old Tuberculin) and PPD (Purified Protein Derivative) had a reduced ability to develop cellular reactivity to these antigenic entities in adulthood, whereas early exposure to intact tubercle bacilli failed to induce tolerance and instead brought about sensitization, despite the immaturity of the animals (18, 19).

It was considered possible that this early sensitization by the whole organisms might perhaps arise from a stimulating effect on lymphoid maturation and functional capacity. The adjuvant properties of mycobacteria were indeed well known (20), and although their mechanisms were then and are still today obscure, subsequent work with MER and other tubercle bacillus entities has documented their profound influence on RES-lymphoid morphological and functional development. At the time, however, the intention was to pursue the possibility of inducing specific immunological unresponsiveness to isolated microbial antigens as a means of analyzing the role of given antigen-antibody reactions in various parasitic associations. Preliminary observations in other systems suggested the feasibility of this approach (21), especially in view of the findings that tolerance can be induced against antigens far removed from self provided that the tolerigen is maintained in the tissues (22). It was only an unexpected circumstance which again focused attention on MER, and thereby changed the senior author's research interests in the direction of "nonspecific immunity" and tumor immunology.

IMMUNIZING PROPERTIES OF MER AGAINST TUBERCULOSIS
IN GUINEA PIGS AND AGAINST AN UNRELATED BACTERIAL PATHOGEN

In the mid-1950s, the British Ministry of Supply opened the doors of its biological warfare research establishment at Porton, near Salisbury, to investigators wishing to undertake nonmilitary projects in these excellent facilities. Dr. Wells and the senior author were invited there to repeat in guinea pigs the antituberculosis immunization studies with nonliving vaccines which had been conducted in mice at the Rockefeller Institute.

The invitation was a very attractive one. Mice represent an unsatisfactory host model of tuberculosis in man, but few institutions could afford to provide the necessary numbers of guinea pigs, a more suitable model animal, for systematic vaccination studies. Porton had an excellent guinea pig colony, and we accordingly availed ourselves of the generous offer to study in the guinea pig the protective immunogenicity of living and killed tubercle bacilli, methanol extracts, and MER against i.p., i.m. and inhalation infection with virulent tubercle bacilli, in addition to the basic investigations on immunological tolerance which were under way at Oxford.

The results of the guinea pig experiments were unambiguous (13, 23, 24). As had been reported by most previous investigators, and has since been confirmed repeatedly, absolute protection could not be elicited against infection with numbers of bacilli sufficient to lead to progressive, fatal disease in a majority of control animals within several months. However, immunization with living BCG did bring about a considerable slowing of the course of infection, and intact phenolized organisms were equally effective at optimal dosage. In many, though not all, of the experiments, the methanolic bacillary extract was also somewhat immunogenic. MER, on the other hand, was at least as effective as living BCG, and occasionally somewhat more so; it evoked only a slight degree of tuberculin hypersensitivity; it was well tolerated, even i.p., at optimally effective dosages; and it acted synergistically with subeffective amounts of the extracts.

From this confirmation of the earlier data obtained in mice, MER emerged as a reliable, safe and effective antituberculosis vaccine, possessing also the considerable advantage of sensitizing only minimally to tuberculin.

The Porton studies would have brought to an end our further basic interest in MER, had it not been for an unforseen occurrence which demonstrated its ability to protect against an unreiated microbial pathogen as well.

Guinea pigs require a constant source of vitamin C in their diet, and in England this is usually provided by fresh cabbage. The Englishman's predilection for this delicacy in shared by another British creature, the wild wood pigeon. These birds carry endemically *Pasteurella pseudotuberculosis,* a gram-negative bacterium highly virulent for many animals, including guinea pigs, and causing visceral lesions superficially resembling those of disseminated tuberculosis. Taxonomically and, as far as is known, antigenically, *P. pseudotuberculosis* is, however, unrelated to the mycobacteria.

The number of heavily infected wood pigeons increases each year with the advance of the seasons, and by late autumn numbers of unusually slow flying birds can be seen in many flocks. Slow flyers which are shot down selectively and examined are found to have considerable disease. In the usual epidemic pattern, the more heavily infected birds succumb rapidly during the first cold spells of winter, reducing the reservoir of infection. In the winter of 1956–57, however, the number of diseased birds which survived late was sufficient to cause extensive contamination of the cabbage with which the Porton guinea pigs were supplied, with the result that an extensive epidemic of *P. pseudotuberculosis* broke out among these animals. At its height, several hundred guinea pigs perished daily, including most of the animals which had been immunized some weeks previously in anticipation of experimental tuberculosis infection. To our surprise, however, guinea pigs which had been given 0.5 to 1.5 mg MER proved almost wholly immune to the pasteurella epidemic which decimated the other animals housed in the same rooms.

We were thus suddenly faced with the observation that a bacterial material derived from one type of organism could protect against lethal infection by another in a "natural" epidemiologic circumstance, and our attention was turned perforce to the nonspecific immunogenic potential of MER.

THE QUESTION OF THE SPECIFICITY OF ACQUIRED ANTIMICROBIAL PROTECTION

The topic of the specificity of microbially induced states of heightened resistance to infection was just then coming into new focus. The elegant studies of Westphal and his associates (25) had recently shown that the endotoxin lipopolysaccharides (LPS) of gram-negative bacteria could lower or elevate, often bimodally within a matter of hours or days, the resistance of animals against microbial pathogens of apparently unrelated antigenicity, and it had also been reported that pretreatment with LPS could heighten immunological responsiveness to certain entirely distinct antigens (26). We, too, had already observed that coadministration of typhoid LPS increased the antituberculosis immunogenicity of methanol extracts in mice (11, 27). Egg yolk sphingomyelin (which could have been contaminated with LPS) appeared to elicit a similar effect (11), as did commercial pertussis vaccine (27). The latter agent, moreover, was found to be capable by itself of enlarging resistance to experimental tuberculosis (28) and of exerting a variety of nonspecifically directed effects on host responsiveness (29). The question of what is specific and what nonspecific in acquired resistance to tuberculosis and other infectious diseases, thus suddenly took on cogency.

Elements of nonspecificity in host-pathogen interactions were already recognized early after the establishment of the germ theory of disease (30, 31)*, but it was not until nonspecific resistance effects were associated with certain at least partially characterized microbial entities active at low concentrations that this aspect of immunity compelled serious consideration. The long and conspicuous neglect of nonspecific resistance factors as significant components of host immunity originated in the protracted and bitter conceptual struggle which preceded the final establishment of microorganisms as the causative agents of many diseases.

By the latter half of the 19th century, the main line of argument was drawn between the proponents of individually specific, clearly definable,

---

* The reader will find of special interest the extensive reviews prepared by Mrs. Helen Nauts and her colleagues of the New York Cancer Research Institute (32, 33) of the extensive early literature dealing with instances of seeming cure or amelioration of neoplastic and other diseases following an infectious disease episode. These reviews also report early experimental experiences with "Coley's toxin" and other microbial products as therapeutic agents in malignant diseases. Although the early observations and experiments which make up this literature fail in most instances to meet currently accepted standards of controlled examination and interpretation, they leave a persuasive impression that contact with certain microorganisms can indeed effect host responses to other parasites, including neoplastic ones. (For a discussion of the view of neoplastic cells as parasites, see the Preface and Introduction to this volume.) A scientific foundation for this impression has been created more recently, as described in this essay.

living microbial agents as the initiators of infectious diseases and those who denied causality to the demonstrated presence of bacteria in pathologic material, or postulated a reverse association: the disease state produces the microbial manifestations. The victorious defenders of the germ theory of disease extended their concept of specificity to states of acquired immunity as well, and also left their mark in a rigidly monomorphic view of microbial structure which persisted for decades.

A hard position on specificity in all aspects of the biology of bacteria and of their interaction with host organisms was clearly necessary in face of the formidable opposition of a scientific establishment which ridiculed microbial causality in natural phenomena (34) and which, to the extent that it regarded microorganisms at all, did so in vague, pleomorphic and often vitalistic terms. Thus, the concept of specific pathogenicity and immunogenicity became an increasingly doctrinal part of the developing germ theory following the forceful and persuasive defense of the specificity of infectious diseases by Bretonneau in the early 19th century (35, 36).

The emphasis on specificity was strengthened by the early success of specific immunization which followed the final acceptance of Koch's Postulates as the operative definition of the germ theory of disease in the last decade of the 19th century. When it became apparent that immunization-induced heightened immunity, as well as the acquired immunity manifested in survivors of frank disease, could be attributed frequently to the induction of specific antibodies (and, as was recognized later, of specifically sensitized cells of the reticuloendothelial-lymphoid system), a direct semantic as well as conceptual association between acquired immunity or resistance, specificity and antibodies (and specifically sensitized cells) became unavoidable. Conversely and by default, nonspecificity became associated with mechanisms other than antibodies or specifically sensitized cells. A corollary association was equally inescapable: specific antibody mechanisms of immunity are both definable and successful, and are therefore of major importance; in contrast, nonspecific ones are vague and not clearly associated with successful protection, and are therefore of minor importance. Although the existence of nonspecific factors in native (or "natural") resistance was not as such seriously attacked, their function in the total ability of organisms to withstand infection was largely ignored, and very little allowance was made for their participation in the mechanisms of the immunity acquired by preceding contact with microorganisms.

172   D. W. WEISS AND D. J. YASHPHE

The new body of information developing in the 1950s, which pointed to a large area of lability in the concepts of host-parasite specificity, placed not only the logic of these semantic associations into question, but the very meaning of the terms "specific" and "nonspecific." These newer data could not be dismissed easily because they were based on readily reproducible experiments with delimited bacterial entities. Moreover, many of the early and convincing observations were made in the system of experimental tuberculosis, considered twenty years ago, as it still is by many investigators today, as a critical model of the nature and complexities of chronic host-parasite associations. Thus, the findings of Weiss and Dubos that pretreatment with nonmycobacterial agents could protect against mycobacterial infection were repeated by other workers in Dr. Dubos' laboratories (28, 37) and by investigators elsewhere (38, 39). Conversely, the guinea pig-pasteurella observations at Porton were supported by a number of other studies showing that whole tubercle bacilli and certain derivatives, including the residues of methanol extractions, could indeed induce heightened resistance to other bacterial pathogens (14, 40, 41). It would appear most unlikely that the broad spectrum of nonspecific immunogenicity which was subsequently shown for mycobacteria can be ascribed to the presence of cross-reactive antigens in the challenge organisms. It must be noted, however, that mycobacteria do share common antigens with at least some taxonomically distant microorganism (42) and an element of specific immunological stimulation in "nonspecific" immunity elicited by tubercle bacilli cannot be ruled out in all instances.

The new observations on nonspecific immunogenicity now posed a number of unavoidable and central questions: Is the protection against tuberculosis elicited by tubercle bacillus substances perhaps based on the same, nonspecific mechanisms responsible for their protective action against other infections? Do specific antibodies and sensitized lymphoid and macrophagic cells perhaps play only a minor role, or no role at all, in the acquired immunity to tubercle bacilli which results from a specific previous contact? On the other hand, are the resistance bestowed against tuberculosis by unrelated agents and the nonspecific protective capacity of the tubercle bacillus perhaps due to a nonspecific stimulation of specific mechanisms, including immunological ones? It appeared questionable, moreover, whether specificity could always be equated with immunological responsiveness in the classic sense of antibody and sensitized cell formation; enzymatic, hormonal, and other highly specific biological mechanisms could also well be imagined to play decisive roles in highly specific defense reactions.*

The unexpected finding that MER protected against an unrelated pathogen, *P. pseudotuberculosis*, under epidemiological circumstances, thus focused our attention on a new and much wider interest, nonspecificity in infectious disease relationships. When explorative experiments indicated that MER could also protect mice against a strain of *Pasteurella pestis* (43) and against other bacterial infections, it was decided to investigate more systematically the extent and parameters of its nonspecific protective capabilities, with the aim of defining nonspecific resistance as a significant biological phenomenon extending beyond the bacterial endotoxins and gram-negative infections. For a number of reasons, MER appeared to be an attractive test substance for a model study.

PREPARATION OF MER AND SOME OF ITS PROPERTIES

Preparation. Because MER is a crude bacterial fraction, and because there are as yet no chemical or other correlative tests of its nonspecific biological activities, special care has been given to standardizing its preparation.

In most of the studies subsequent to the guinea pig tuberculosis experiments at Porton, the source organisms were two BCG-Phipps strains, and preparation has been by very similar protocols, varying slightly only in regard to the time sequence of methanol extraction. Batches made in recent years have always been started from lyophilized BCG cultures. The organisms are grown as pellicles for several weeks, usually four, on Bacto-Dubos medium (Difco Laboratories, Inc., Detroit) without Tween

---

* The terms "specific" and "nonspecific" should, accordingly, be employed only to indicate the direction of effects in symbiotic relationships, including host-parasite associations in infectious diseases, without any bias as to mechanism, and it is in this light that the words will be used here. Thus, "specific" resistance or immunity will describe conditions of refractoriness to disease and disease agents induced by preceding experience with the causative or related agents; and "nonspecific" resistance or immunity to those accruing from experience with unrelated factors. The terms "homologous" and "heterologous" are perhaps more satisfactory alternatives for "specific" and "nonspecific," respectively (44), and will also be employed in this synonymous sense. "Resistance" and "immunity" will be used interchangeably, in the absence of a generally accepted convention associating the terms with either the mechanism or the degree of ability to withstand.

(polyoxyethylene sorbitan mono-oleate), but with the addition of 1.5% glycerol. The cultures are then killed by contact with 2% phenol for 18 to 24 hr at room temperature. The phenol is removed by repeated washings of the pellicular mass placed in a cheese-cloth filter, first with distilled water and then with cold acetone. Some of the acetone-soluble lipids, which possess toxic properties, are thus removed. The bacillary mass is then air dried at room temperature, ground with mortar and pestle*, and stored over a desiccant at 4 C until used.

Methanol extraction is performed with repeated quantities of fresh absolute methanol, in a flask fitted with a reflux condenser and placed in a 56 C water bath. The extraction mixture is continuously agitated by means of a magnetic stirrer. After each period of extraction, the hot alcohol is decanted, and a new quantity added. After the last extraction, the residue is suspended in a small quantity of acetone, air-dried, ground with mortar and pestle, and stored in the cold over a desiccant. A typical protocol of MER preparation is shown in Fig. 1.

To make a suspension of MER, the desired amount is ground in a mortar into a paste, employing very small quantities' of pyrogen-free aqueous diluent. After thorough grinding, the paste is transferred to a small glass vessel with more diluent and stirred for 5 to 10 min at high speed in a VirTis stirrer; the mixture is then brought to the required volume with the remaining diluent.

Physical properties. Aqueous suspensions of MER are very unstable, and syringes or pipets should be filled with only the amount to be injected or transferred in a single dose, to prevent uneven distribution due to settling out of the larger particles.

In its dry state, MER has been stored in the cold for as long as five years without evidence of decreased nonspecific protective and immunological activity. It has also been maintained at 4 C for several months in aqueous suspension and in a stabilizing agent provided by Merk & Co.** without decrease of activity. MER in coarse aqueous suspension appears to be stable to heating for 10 to 15 min at 70 C, and there is indication that it resists even higher temperatures.

It may be that the biological activities of MER are dependent at least

---

* The dry bacillary powder, and also MER, are handled only in a hood under negative pressure, to prevent accidental inhalation of the fine, dustlike material.
** This agent consists of carboxymethyl cellulose, polysorbate 80, and benzyl alcohol, in a saline base.

Day	Procedure
1	Weigh out 3.5 g phenol-killed, acetone-washed, dried BCG bacillary powder. Grind finely with mortar and pestle. Place in extraction flask, and add 500 ml absolute anhydrous methanol. Extract for 6 to 8 hr at 55 to 56 C. Permit to stand at room temperature overnight.
2	Continue hot extraction for 6 to 8 hr. Decant methanol and add 500 ml fresh methanol. Permit to stand at room temperature overnight.
3	Continue hot extraction for 6 to 8 hr. Permit to stand at room temperature overnight.
4	Continue hot extraction for 6 to 8 hr. Decant 250 ml methanol and add 250 ml fresh methanol. Permit to stand at room temperature overnight.
5	Continue hot extraction for 6 to 8 hr. Permit to stand at room temperature for 48 hr.
7	Continue hot extraction for 6 to 8 hr. Permit to stand at room temperature overnight.
8	Continue hot extraction for 6 to 8 hr. Decant 250 ml methanol and add 250 ml fresh methanol. Permit to stand at room temperature overnight.
9	Continue hot extraction for 4 to 6 hr. Decant all the methanol, and transfer the bacterial residue to a crystallizing dish. With a porcelain spatula make a paste of the residue with pure acetone, and add enough acetone to cover. Permit the residue to dry completely out of the acetone, covering the dish with one or two layers of sterile cheesecloth and placing it in a sterile hood. (12 to 36 hr of drying is sufficient. If the mass is not dry after 12 hr, a small amount of acetone may be added again to disperse it and it is permitted to dry again.)

The MER is then ground in a mortar and pestle in the hood, transferred to sterile bottles, weighed and stored at 4 C in a desiccator over a drying agent.

All utensils and containers with which MER comes into contact are washed thoroughly, rinsed 20 times with deionized, pyrogen-free water and sterilized in a hot oven.

FIG. 1.   Preparation of MER.

in part on critical aspects of its physical state. Attempts in our laboratories and at the Merck Research Institute (D. E. Wolf, personal communication) to obtain active subfractions by means of further extraction with chloroform, ether, acetone and ethyl alcohol, alone and in mixtures, yielded extracts which were only sporadically active in the standard Klebsiella protection assay (described below), and usually to a lower degree than the parent material. In contrast, the particulate residues of these further extractions almost always showed activity. Sonic disruption of MER destroyed activity at the point where the substance lost its particulate nature.

The chemical determinants of MER activity are unknown. It may not be unreasonable to assume that a lipopolysaccharide moiety [perhaps related to the mycolic acid-glycopeptide compounds which possess classical adjuvant activity (45, 46)] plays an active role (47), as is the case with at least some other nonspecifically active bacterial substances, but there is no direct evidence for this supposition. It must be emphasized that the biological activities of MER are both quantitatively and qualitatively decidedly distinct in many respects from those manifested by the gram-negative bacterial endotoxin LPS and the other known agents capable of inducing heterologous resistance and immunological effects, including other mycobacterial preparations. If LPS are involved in MER activity, they must, accordingly, either be molecules with very unique properties, or act in association with other molecular entities.

It is possible that native components of the tubercle bacillus are exposed or altered, or both, in the process of MER preparation, providing moieties with different biological potential. Thus, for example, it has been suggested by Ribi that the exposure of constituents lining the interior of the bacterial cell wall, brought about by certain fractionation procedures, is responsible for the exceptionally high homologous immunizing properties of certain tubercle bacillus fractions (48).

Attempts at the chemical isolation and characterization of MER active principle(s) are now being planned (M. Tishler, personal communication), with special attention to the physicochemical attributes of the material.

Biological properties. MER sensitizes to tuberculoproteins, but to a much lesser extent than intact living or inactivated BCG organisms (13).

MER is well tolerated by young adult mice in amounts up to 1.0 to 1.5 mg dry wt, even when injected i.p., and by guinea pigs in considerably larger doses. In terms of its effects on weight gain, general behavior, appearance of fur, and gross neurologic function, MER is better accepted than whole phenolized BCG in equal quantities (24).

When injected s.c. into mice or guinea pigs, granulomas develop locally. These go on to limited tubercle formation and may break through the skin. Healing of the local lesions is slow, and follows the typical course of tubercles induced by other nonliving mycobacterial entities.

Following i.p. administration, the material is seen for many months in small, opaque nodules scattered over the omentum, mesenteries, and surface of the viscera. These nodules also resemble tubercles histologically. Histological examination of other organs has revealed no signs of granuloma formation or other damage induced by MER for periods of up to several months following i.p. administration of 0.5 to 1.0 mg: the heart, lungs, kidneys, liver, small intestine and pancreas of treated mice appear to be unaffected, except for an occasional, limited appearance of inflammatory fat tissue in the pancreas. This change in the pancreas might be ascribed to the immediate proximity of a small mesenteric tubercle.

More extensive studies are now under way at the National Cancer Institute of the USPHS on possibly more occult toxic effects of MER in rodents, rabbits and dogs. As a derivative of inactivated, attenuated tubercle bacilli, it is very unlikely, however, that MER will be found to cause appreciable systemic injury at dosage levels required to elicit effects on immunity.

Active lots of MER which have been examined for pyrogenicity in rabbits and dogs were found to be free of pyrogenic properties.

The optimal dose of MER for mice spans the same dose range in all the models of nonspecific protection and immunological modulation which have been studied. The precise quantity varies with batch and experiment from 0.25 to 1.0 mg, but is most commonly in the vicinity of 0.5 mg given once or twice prior to, and sometimes after, challenge. In the two test systems using guinea pigs in which MER was employed, protection against tuberculous infection and induction of delayed hypersensitivity to protein-hapten conjugates (see below), the optimum doses were similar to those for mice. A body weight-dosage relationship thus does not appear to exist; this is not necessarily surprising for a long-retained bacterial entity which probably induces complex and interacting responses in the host, some of which may perpetuate themselves for considerable periods of time once they are begun, and partly without further contribution by the initiating agent.

Virtually every batch of MER prepared by the standard procedure has been active in the Klebsiella protection test, although batches with uncommonly high or with more limited capacity have occasionally been produced. Activity in the Klebsiella assay appears to be a good indication of efficacy in at least some of the other protection and immunological response systems, but no attempt has been made as yet to subject all lots of MER systematically to every test in which the various preparations have been found active.

Both the s.c. and the i.p. routes of MER administration have proven effective in a number of test systems, but in at least some instances, the latter is more consistently reliable and has, accordingly, been the preferred method in many of the mouse experiments. Even where s.c. injection of MER does elicit nonspecific effects, somewhat larger quantities are at times required to yield results similar to those obtained by i.p. treatment. Administration by both routes is efficacious in heightening resistance to some pathogenic cells and in modifying the response to some antigens, even when challenge is by another portal of entry; but, as will be described later, challenge is preferentially by the same route as MER treatment to obtain marked effects in other test systems.

In the guinea pig-protein-DNP conjugate sensitization system described below, i.c. administration of MER was found to be effective as well.

NONSPECIFIC ANTIMICROBIAL ACTIVITY OF MER

Extensive experiments conducted in the laboratories of the Department of Bacteriology and Immunology of the University of California in Berkeley, the Merck Research Institute in Rahway, New Jersey and Parke, Davis & Co. in Detroit revealed MER to be capable of eliciting some degree of heightened resistance in mice against subsequent challenge with every bacterial pathogen tested (44). These included several strains of *Klebsiella pneumoniae* and *Staphylococcus aureus,* an attenuated strain of *Pasteurella pestis* capable of causing death when given in large numbers and strains of *Streptococcus pyogenes, Diplococcus pneumoniae, Proteus mirabilis, Pseudomonas aeruginosa* and *Salmonella typhimurium.*

Protection was manifested even against very strong challenge, as great as 18 to 20 LD_{50} of *Klebsiella pneumoniae**, for example, and appeared to reach a peak within 24 hr after administration of MER. (It is noted, as described below, that considerably longer time intervals between MER treatment and challenge are required for optimum effects in a number of tumor systems, and that in some instances maximum effects are elicited when treatment is given after challenge.) Heightened resistance was discernible even when MER was given only several hours prior to, or at the time of, infection. A negative phase of reduced resistance after injection of MER was never observed within the range of quantities employed, 0.1 to 1.5 mg dry wt. The state of heightened resistance was

---
* Protection against experimental Klebsiella infection is now used as a standard bioassay for MER activity. Active lots of the material, given i.p. in quantities of 0.25 to 1.0 mg, three to seven days prior to infection, protect at least 60% of outbred young adult albino mice against 3 to 5 LD_{50} of i.p. administered *K. pneumoniae.*

consistently evident for at least 10 days, though occasionally at a reduced level at the longer intervals, and was frequently manifested even after several weeks to months. Against some of the pathogens, as little as 0.2 mg MER induced significant protection, whereas against others 0.5 to 1.0 mg were necessary. Living BCG (0.5-ml quantities of 1/5 to 1/50 dilutions of young cultures) was consistently ineffective in these studies.

The protective effect of MER was more apparent in female than in male mice.

Administration of MER to breeding females markedly reduced the incidence of an endemic viral pneumonitis among their offspring, even those born nearly a year after treatment of the mothers, and increased the number of litters carried to term late after treatment (in the 11th post-treatment month).

NONSPECIFIC ANTITUMOR ACTIVITY OF MER

In the summer of 1958, the senior author attended a meeting in Freiburg, Germany, devoted to the nonspecific resistance effects elicited by microbial fractions. In the course of an informal discussion on the possible evolutionary functions of the vertebrate immunological apparatus, the suggestion was voiced that the immune response in its classical manifestations may have developed at the level of the primitive vertebrates, where true neoplasia seems to make its first phylogenetic appearance, as a new, surveillance mechanism to protect the individual from his own neoplastic cells. At the same meeting, Benacceraf presented the findings of a series of experiments, subsequently published (49) which showed that living BCG could increase the resistance of mice against homografts of tumor cells. Upon returning to Berkeley, the senior author suggested to Dr. K. B. DeOme of the Cancer Research Genetics Laboratory of the University of California the desirability of testing the MER fraction against syngeneic tumor transplants, on the grounds that a broadly active resistance stimulator might have activity against neoplastic as well as against microbial pathogens.

Dr. DeOme pointed out the weakness of this suggestion, that it was based on two suppositions for which evidence was lacking: One, that the nonspecific protective activities of MER were indeed the outcome of effects exerted on immunological function; and two, that neoplastic cells of autochthonous origin are, in fact, recognized as antigenically distinct by their host. This latter principle was supported at the time only by the still preliminary work of Foley (50) and of Prehn and Main

(51), showing that mouse sarcomas induced by chemical carcinogens are immunogenic in the isogenic animal. These findings were then not yet generally accepted as creating a valid basis for the special immunology of neoplastic tissues.

The early development of tumor immunology as a legitimate discipline had been marked by prematurely high expectations and hopes, but it was subsequently recognized that the apparent successes of earlier investigators represented artifacts. The consequent disappointment led to the equally unbalanced view, still rather prevalent in 1958, that investigators who viewed neoplasia in immunological terms were, at best, wishful dreamers sadly lacking in objectivity.

From the beginning of oncology as an experimental study, the expectation had been held that certain immune reactions are directed specifically against cancer cells, and that such reactions could be extended towards therapeutic goals. The basis of this view was simple, and can be considered essentially correct today: Neoplastic cells differ from analogous normal ones in behavior and appearance; such differences must be based, ultimately, on differences in macromolecular composition or arrangement; and deviations in such composition or arrangement are likely to lead to new antigenic properties. The difficulty lay with the attempt to provide experimental evidence in support of this hypothesis. In spite of Woglom's classic warning that "far too large a proportion of cancer immunity experiments are merely ridiculous, for few investigators seem to realize that cancer research is a discipline requiring some apprenticeship, and that not everyone with an inoculating needle and a dozen white mice can plunge in and emerge with a discovery" (52), numerous workers conducted studies in which little effort was made to distinguish supposed tumor-specific immune phenomena from homograft reactivity in general. When the principles governing the transplantability of normal tissues came to be more fully recognized, virtually the entire body of information on "tumor immunology" had to be discarded as proving no more than that animals can react immunologically to antigens possessed by individuals of another genotype. Only after Foley (50), Prehn (51), the Kleins (53, 54) and, subsequently, many other groups had carefully demonstrated the isogenicity of tumor donor and test animals in various systems, was a valid foundation for tumor immunology slowly created.

In the late 1950s, however, the general climate of opinion on tumor immunology was still a largely pessimistic one, and although the demonstrations of the specific immunogenicity of some carcinogen-induced tumors appeared incontrovertible, it was generally still held that spontaneously arising tumors are not uniquely antigenic.

Nonetheless, Dr. DeOme decided to risk seven BALB/c mice on an experiment. Three of these were given MER, four served as saline controls, and all were then implanted with an isogenic, spontaneously arisen uterine sarcoma. No tumor growth occurred in the three MER-treated mice. A repeat experiment with 15 animals, and a subsequent one conducted by Dr. DeOme himself with 36, gave identical findings. The random choice of this test tumor was fortunate, because, as became evident later, few mouse neoplasms can be so decisively protected against by MER pretreatment as this BALB/c sarcoma.

These initial observations of the effects of MER in an isogeneic tumor model led the senior author into three avenues of investigation: A descriptive analysis of the effects of MER on resistance to isogenic and autochthonous neoplastic cells; an endeavor to understand the mode of action of MER, with emphasis on a determination of its effects on humoral and cellular immune responses against known antigens; and a study of the occurrence and nature of antigenic properties associated with the neoplastic state.

Along the latter line of work, attention was focused on the supposedly nonantigenic spontaneous mammary carcinomas of mice, and it was successfully demonstrated that these tumors are, in effect, recognized as antigenic by the autochthonous and isogenic animal, provided that the hosts are not rendered specifically unresponsive to mammary tumor virus (MTV)-associated antigens on the cell surface as a result of exposure to the virus in early life (55–58). Furthermore, a proportion of these mammary carcinomas carry antigens not related to the presence of the etiologic MTV, and are reacted against even by mice tolerant to the agent (57, 59, 60). The actuality and biologic characterization of the antigenicity of these tumors was corroborated by other workers, and the tumor-associated antigenicity (for an explanation of the emphasis on the term "tumor-associated," and avoidance of the term "tumor specific," see references 61, 62) of most, if not all, experimental and spontaneous neoplasms of animals and man is firmly established today (54, 63). Progressive neoplasia has thus come to be viewed as the consequence, at least in part, of immunological deficiency or aberration.

The results of experiments along the two former pathways of research are discussed below.

Effects of MER on the development of various tumor isografts in mice. In an initial series of screening experiments, MER was given to young adult mice before or after challenge with isografts of several spontaneously arisen or induced solid tumors: the BALB/c uterine sarcoma; a hepatoma which developed in C3H mice treated with carbon tetrachloride; a spontaneous RIII mammary adenocarcinoma; a spontaneous C3H osteogenic sarcoma; several methylcholanthrene-induced BALB/c fibrosarcomas; a spontaneous DBA/2 fibrosarcoma; and a spontaneous C57Bl myeloid leukemia in solid form (64, 65).

Against one of the induced fibrosarcomas and against the spontaneous one, MER petreatment in the quantities used (0.5 to 1.0 mg) at times induced apparently greater susceptibility, i.e., enhanced growth of the isografts; living and phenol-killed BCG, which were tested as well against the one carcinogen-induced tumor, elicited a similar effect. No effect was evinced by MER vis-à-vis the C57Bl myeloid leukemia, whereas pretreatment with living BCG did afford a degree of heightened resistance against this tumor. In all other instances, MER pretreatment consistently bestowed heightened resistance, and usually to a greater extent than did pretreatment with living or killed BCG or with methanol extract. The heightened refractoriness was evidenced either by a reduction in the number of animals developing progressively growing tumors, or by an increased incidence of regressions, or, most commonly, by a retarded tumor growth rate. Although pretreatment was more potent in most cases, injection of MER after tumor implantation was usually at least somewhat effective and, in some models, considerably so. In most experiments, MER was administered i.p. but the s.c. route was also found to be at least partially satisfactory when employed. The experimental parameters necessary to demonstrate maximal protective effects varied somewhat from system to system, but as in the antimicrobial pathogen models, optimum activity was always within a dose range of 0.25 to 1.0 mg MER given by single or double injection. MER pretreatment was efficacious even when several months elapsed between administration and tumor challenge; there was a definite impression of a lesser efficacy when challenge was earlier than two weeks after treatment.

MER pretreatment did not cause a rejection of first or second set skin isografts, thus indicating that the effects elicited against tumor isografts could not be ascribed to a residual heterozygosis of isoantigenic characteristics.

These experiments, which have been repeated numerous times with very similar results in large numbers of mice, thus revealed MER to be a strong modulator of resistance against tumor isografts, usually heightening resistance, but on occasion stimulating accelerated tumor growth. This two-directional potential of MER nonspecific immune stimulation resembles the potentially diverse effects of specific immunization with living or inactivated tumor tissue, which may also be manifested by either increased resistance to subsequent tumor challenge, or by increased susceptibility, i.e., immunological enhancement (66–68). It thus appeared of primary importance to determine, if possible, the parameters of MER administration, with and without accompanying' specific immunization, which direct the immune response towards heightened resistance and those which direct it towards heightened susceptibility to the neoplastic cells. In immunological terms, this question could be restated as follows: Under which conditions does MER treatment modulate the immune response against tumor-associated antigens in the direction of cellular (and perhaps also macroglobulin) reactivity, and under which in the direction of IgG antibodies, some of which have enhancing activity?

Although humoral antibodies are undoubtedly of significance in resistance to certain microbial parasites, perhaps play an ancillary role in the rejection of foreign solid tissues* and (at least some antibodies, most probably those of the IgM type) may by themselves be effective in destroying some leukemic and ascitic cancer cells and incipient metastatic foci, it is generally accepted that it is the cellular component of the immune response which is largely responsible for immunological surveillance against neoplastic cells and for resistance against many pathogenic microorganisms.

Two lines of investigation were initiated to provide information on this critical point: an analysis of the parameters of MER influence on cellular and humoral immune responsiveness to defined antigens, and a more systematic study of its resistance-modulating activities against two categories of neoplasms in mice. For the latter purpose, one type of solid and one of leukemic neoplasm were chosen, spontaneous mammary carcinomas in C3H and BALB/c animals and radiation-virus-induced leukemia in the C57Bl/6 strain.

Effects of MER on spontaneous mammary carcinomas of C3H and

---

* It has recently been suggested by Harris and Harris (personal communication) that IgG_2 antibodies may play an important role in the rejection of foreign skin grafts.

BALB/c mice. 1) Primary tumor development in the autochthonous host: C3H females were given several i.p. injections of MER during the first several months of life, up to a total of 2.5 to 5.0 mg, and were then employed as breeding animals under the standard conditions of the Cancer Research Genetics Laboratory breeding colony. They, and a parallel control group which received saline injections, were observed periodically for 18 months for onset of gross (palpable) mammary tumors.

The development of the tumors was retarded and reduced in the MER-treated mice (69). In a second experiment, C3H females were given two injections i.p., at two and five months of age, of either saline only, living BCG (0.5 ml of a 1/25 dilution of an eight-day-old liquid animals receiving the smallest amount of MER, tumor onset was signif-icantly delayed as compared with the controls, whereas animals given ficantly delayed as compared with the controls, whereas animals given the largest quantity of MER or living BCG showed a clearly accelerated tumor development.

These findings thus again indicated that significant protection can be elicited against neoplastic cells, even where these develop spontaneously in the primary host, provided that the correct parameters of MER treat-ment are found—and these may be narrow.

2) Development of preneoplastic hyperplastic alveolar nodules: It has been shown by the extensive experiments of DeOme, Bern and Nandi (70) that spontaneous mammary carcinomas of mice infected with MTV do not arise directly from normal mammary parenchyma, but rather from hyperplastic alveolar nodules (HAN). These structures are morphologically identical with normal mammary gland in the lobular alveolar state of late pregnancy and lactation, but they are also seen in certain strains of mice after the remaining gland has regressed to the ductile form, typical of virgin females, with the cessation of lactation. The nodules also appear in virgin females of some strains late in life, and their appearance can be hastened by hormonal manipulation as well as by pregnancy. As precursors of frank mammary carcinomas, the HAN are defined as preneoplastic lesions; their biological behavior does not fall into the category of true neoplasia, but is deviant from that of normal mammary tissue in a number of respects.

Experiments were undertaken to ascertain whether MER treatment can influence the development of the preneoplastic HAN in young C3H mice hormonally stimulated by the implantation of several isogenic pituitaries or by injection of estrogen and deoxycorticosterone (69). The results showed a clear and marked protective effect by MER on HAN development.

Preliminary studies (D. W. Weiss, unpublished results) have also indicated that MER treatment may slow the further transformation of outgrowths of HAN to full-fledged mammary carcinomas, but the effect seen in these exploratory experiments appeared to be a more modest one.

3) Development of mammary carcinoma isografts: A large number of experiments have been conducted with mammary tumor isografts, employing tumors infected with MTV both in similarly infected C3H and BALB /cfC3H animals and in uninfected mice of the same genotype (C3Hf and BALB/c). Parallel studies have been carried out with isografts of mammary tumors arising in animals of MTV-free strains which had been stimulated hormonally for prolonged periods of time. Many of these studies are still in progress, but a pattern of MER effects has begun to emerge.

Intraperitoneal or s.c. pretreatment with MER alone, in quantities ranging from 0.5 to 2.0 mg, bestowed on occasion heightened resistance against the tumor isografts, but sometimes accelerated tumor growth instead (65, 71).* Preliminary experiments suggest that with still smaller amounts of MER, however, the much more usual effect is increased resistance and that enhancement is elicited very rarely. Similarly, specific immunization with tumor cells alone sometimes leads to heightened resisatnce, but not infrequently, especially in the case of MTV-free BALB/c mice immunized with MTV-free mammary carcinomas, gives rise to accelerated tumor progression, which appears to be classical immunological enhancement (72). [The tendency of mammary carcinomas of mice to undergo enhancement, perhaps related to the circumstances that at least one of the strong tumor-associated antigens is organ-specific to the mammary gland and

---

* *Note added in proof*: The enhanced growth of some tumors which is induced by pretreatment with MER may not, in fact, always represent classical immunological enhancement mediated by free, specific antibodies. It may instead reflect antigenic competition or preemption by the MER fraction which is itself immunogenic, or may accrue from the nonspecific lowering of general inflammatory reactivity and of the movement of immunologically potent cells to other inflammatory foci, such as occur in the vicinity of tumor implants, which can be brought about by the tissue deposition of mycobacterial entities (G.L. Asherson, personal communication.)

that organ-specific antigens may have a unique penchant for directing immune responses towards enhancement, has been discussed elsewhere (61).] On the other hand, in animals given dual pretreatment (MER plus specific immunization with living or inactivated tumor cells), this tendency to undergo enhancement is consistently aborted: the mice do not show accelerated tumor development, but usually display some degree of heightened resistance.

When MER was administered s.c. in one or several distal sites after a tumor isograft had already been established, the survival times of the animals were frequently increased and tumor growth was occasionally retarded; at times, however, no effects were elicited on tumor development (I. Eron et al., submitted for publication). When, however, MER treatment was combined with therapeutic local irradiation or with chemotherapy (methotrexate, cyclophosphamide, 5-FU and 6-MP were the agents most commonly employed), or with both irradiation and chemotherapy, a synergistic slowing of tumor growth was evident in many instances and, again, enhancement was not encountered (I. Eron et al., submitted for publication). Injection of MER directly adjacent to the s.c. growing tumor seemed ineffective in altering resistance. [This observation is in contrast to the findings of Rapp et al. (73) with living BCG in an inbred guinea pig-hepatoma system: both local and distal tumor foci regress when BCG is injected directly into one tumor focus, and efficacy appears dependent on the direct contact between neoplastic cells and the vaccine. Possible explanations for these seemingly divergent observations are discussed elsewhere (74).]

In a recently initiated immunotherapy model of investigation, in which a primary or implanted tumor is removed, and local recurrence or metastatic spread is simulated by introducing small numbers of tumor cells into the original tumor area or into the caudal vein, respectively, s.c. MER treatment combined with irradiation or chemotherapy also produced a synergistic heightening of resistance, whereas MER treatment alone was of smaller and less consistent benefit.

Radiation treatment and chemotherapy most probably lead to the death and dissolution of tumor cells, and to a consequent liberation of tumor-associated antigenic moieties. These treatments might thus also resemble, in effect, specific hyperimmunization in terms of an increased exposure of the host to tumor antigens. Why the combination of non-specific immunological stimulation elicited by MER and specific immunization with tumor antigens should lead preferentially to heightened resistance is not understood. It may be that the combined action of specific and nonspecific stimuli affects lymphoid cells in a manner permitting them to act in cellular immune reactions, but disfavoring the release of IgG antibodies. Such lymphoid cells may also be more resistant to radiation and chemotherapy, both factors which reduce immunological reactivity, and may continue to function as effector cells but without having regained their antibody-synthesizing capacity. Whatever the explanation, it appears from these models that combined immuno- and chemotherapy, together with therapeutic irradiation where this is applicable, may have synergistic beneficial effects in attacking tumor cell populations remaining after surgery.

Experiments are under way to determine quantitatively the ability of MER to counteract the immunosuppressive effects of chemotherapy and irradiation, and it may be that a major benefit of MER therapy lies with the prevention of the destruction of immunological capacity which is brought about by most of the agents used today in cancer therapy. Many investigators have come to look upon such therapy as a two-edged sword, and use of MER or other such agents to avoid the negative aspects of cancer treatment may allow more rigorous treatment schedules to be initiated without thereby eradicating the host's own immunological defenses.

Effects of MER on the development of leukemia induced in C57Bl/6 mice by the radiation-leukemia virus. The test system is that developed by Dr. Nechamah Haran-Ghera of the Weizmann Institute, who collaborated with the authors in these studies (75). The animals are infected with passaged viruses originally derived from the tissues of an isogenic mouse exposed to whole body irradiation, known to activate latent leukemogenic agents in this strain. Injection of the viral suspension is directly into one lobe of the thymus. Some of the passaged viral agents are potently leukemogenic by themselves, whereas others induce a high incidence of leukemias only in hosts in whom immunological ability is reduced after infection by means of whole body irradiation or other treatment. In the present experiments, such immunosuppression was achieved by exposing the animals to 400 r X-irradiation two days after infection. MER treatment was by one or several i.p. injections of 0.5 mg each, before or after exposure to the virus.

When MER was first given 30 days after infection with the more potent agent, and again a second time 10 or 30 days thereafter, a degree of protection was elicited. Fewer animals developed leukemia as of the time of writing (10 months postinfection), and the mean time of leukemia onset as indicated by palpable thymus enlargement was delayed. In the case of the less virulent agent, where whole body irradiation was necessary to potentiate leukemogenic action, the effects were even more marked. Mice treated two or three times with MER at 30-day intervals after infection showed only a 10 and 20% leukemia incidence, respectively, whereas 95% of the control animals developed the disease. However, single treatment with 0.5 mg, 30 or 60 days after infection, or single or double treatment begun before infection or sooner than 30 days thereafter, exerted little or no protective effect (N. Haran-Ghera et al., submitted for publication). It is noted that by 30 days after infection, some leukemic cells already appear, and these have been shown to be antigenic in the isogenic host (76). Thus, the optimum conditions of MER treatment again resemble a combined nonspecific and specific immunological stimulation, with the requirement here that the latter precedes.

Further studies are under way with this model, varying the dosage of MER and the schedules of administration, but the results already obtained show once more that major protective effects can be elicited by this substance, within the correct range of parameters of administration. The determination of the appropriate parameters of intervention with MER, and very likely with other nonspecific stimulators of immunological responsiveness as well, thus clearly emerges as a major concern for future studies, including trials in man. There may be not only species and strain variations but also individual variations within these limits. Their definition in each patient may come to be the single most important factor in future attempts at immunotherapy of neoplastic diseases in man.

Preliminary studies on the effects of MER in cancer patients. We have been exceedingly hesitant to begin human studies with MER, despite the recent initiation of immunotherapy of cancer patients in a number of institutions in Europe, the USA and Africa with living BCG and other immunostimulators, whose immunological activities are less known than those of MER. We consider MER primarily as a model of the biological phenomenon of nonspecific immunogenicity, and although it has proven superior in many of our laboratory studies to living BCG, other mycobacterial fractions, DNA digest provided by Dr. Werner Braun of Rutgers University and other active agents supposedly nonspecific, we have no reason to assume that MER is the most effective substance of this kind which can be found or developed. Rather, it has been our intention to work out in detail, at the laboratory level, the activities of MER as a representative agent, in the hope that the information gained will encourage a systematic search for other and perhaps more powerful immunostimulators.

Furthermore, there is the ever-present danger that any immunologic intervention, whether specific or nonspecific, may lead towards enhancement and a consequent worsening of the patient's condition. The arguments that the prognosis in many forms of cancer is in any event ultimately negative for virtually every patient, and that as many or more individuals might be helped by furthering resistance as might be injured by facilitating enhancement, are not convincing.* Ethical reservations to a precipitous and unguided human study are certainly indicated in the present instance, and especially so if ways can possibly be devised to monitor carefully the ongoing effects of MER in cancer patients, so as to adjust treatment individually in the direction of those compartments of immunological reactivity which are associated with improved resistance.

With these reservations in mind, MER has been given in small quantities to a number of patients during the past several years. In each instance, the patient was in an advanced stage of neoplastic illness, and was a close relative of a physician who requested the treatment as a last-straw attempt. In several cases, the attending doctor believed that some improvement followed administration of MER, but the absence of any controls and the small number of patients make it impossible to obtain even a very limited objective impression.

A systematic, controlled study was initiated several months ago in patients with acute leukemia at Hadassah Hospital, in collaboration with Dr. G. Izak. Leukemic patients were chosen for this exploratory study for a number of reasons, chiefly, that the induction of enhancement is very much less likely to occur in leukemias than in cases of solid tumors: the dispersed neoplastic cells appear to be more susceptible to attack even by free antibodies of molecular classes not usually associated with high cytotoxic capacity, and there seems to be much less of a neutralizing or competitive effect elicited by nondestructive antibodies.

Intracutaneous treatment with MER is begun when patients have entered remission, and all patients are kept on standard maintenance therapy. The

---

* I note that within the ethicolegal framework of Judaism, the value of a single life is infinite. If there is definite statistical probability that, in a given group of patients, a fatal disease process may be accelerated by the same treatment which would help others, such a trial is not lightly permissible. — DWW.

patients are randomized into groups which are given either MER according to different schedules, or a placebo only. The major emphasis in this study is on a continuous determination of the effects of MER on immunological capacity, as measured by a repeatedly performed broad battery of tests for humoral and cellular responses, both primary and secondary, to a large number of test antigens and to the patient's own neoplastic cells.

It is hoped from this investigation to obtain answers to several central questions: Can a clear association be shown between increased immunological capacity in one or another direction, and improved clinical course? Can MER under defined conditions of administration predictably modulate immunological responsiveness in humans (in this case, with leukemic neoplasia) along certain lines? Or is it at least possible, by individually adjusting the parameters of repeated MER application, to modify the immunological responsiveness of the particular patient in desired directions, even after treatment has begun?

It is not improbable that the conditions of MER efficacy and of immunological state may be very different in leukemic patients and in those suffering from other types of neoplasia. Nonetheless, answers to such questions coming from this study will at least point to the possibility of treating patients suffering from other forms of cancer with MER and perhaps other nonspecific immunological stimulants, with a satisfactory degree of safety and with a reasonably clear prediction of some success!

Until information accumulates on the relationship between clinical course and differential immunological ability in the leukemia patients, it has been decided to maintain monthly MER treatment, as long as there is evidence of continued elevation of cellular and IgM reactivity, and to discontinue MER when such reactivity reaches a plateau or when IgG antibody responses increase significantly.

This study has not yet advanced far enough to permit any impression other than that the MER-treated patients are in at least as good a clinical condition after several months as the nontreated ones, with a number of the treated persons living longer than was expected upon their admission.

Studies reported from other laboratories on the antitumor effects elicited by MER. Experiments with MER have been undertaken, or are currently in progress, in several other laboratories, and the results already obtained in several of these studies are cited here briefly.

Esber et al. (15, 16) have studied the effects of a methanol extract and a methanol extraction residue of phenol-killed *M. butyricum* on the reactivity of female Fischer 344/CRL strain rats to sheep red blood cells (SRBC), and of the extract on the response to implants of several transplantable mammary carcinomas. Extracts were found to contain small quantities of discrete bacterial fragments, and it is quite possible, therefore, that their activity is the manifestation of a synergistic effect of the extract with small quantities of the residue, as noted previously (13).

Both agents stimulated antibody production to the SRBC when given prior to, with, or after specific immunization, and the extract effectively inhibited tumor growth, especially when its administration was combined with chemotherapy. Some treatment programs evoked enhancement of the tumor implants, rather than resistance. The time of MER administration relative to subsequent tumor challenge appeared to be an important determinant of whether heightened resistance or enhanced susceptibility resulted from the treatment.

Exploratory studies carried out in collaboration with Dr. Charles Evans at the University of Washington in Seattle (C. A. Evans and D. W. Weiss, unpublished observations) suggested that pretreatment with MER can lower the incidence of papilloma formation and subsequent transformation to frank carcinomas in wild San Juan island rabbits infected experimentally with Shope papilloma virus. However, the initial observations have not yet been confirmed.

Lappé has studied the effects of MER on the development of skin tumors arising in mouse skin isografts exposed to methylcholanthrene (77, 78 and personal communication). Treatment of the graft recipients with MER 15 days prior to implantation resulted in a significant delay of papilloma development and in a significantly lower final incidence of papillomas; moreover, a lower proportion of the papillomas progressed to carcinomas. In some experiments, MER pretreatment increased the incidence of papilloma development in the skin transplants, but even in these instances, a higher proportion of the papillomas regressed than in untreated hosts.

In an exploratory experiment, Old (personal communication) observed a marked protective effect of MER against the development of isografts of a murine leukemia.

Studies on the antitumor protective effects of MER are currently in progress in a number of other academic, commercial and governmental laboratories.*

---

* *Note added in proof*: Slemmer has just reported (79) that treatment with MER

EFFECTS OF MER ON IMMUNOLOGICAL RESPONSIVENESS TO KNOWN
ANTIGENS AND ON RETICULOENDOTHELIAL CLEARANCE FUNCTION

Effects of MER on reticuloendothelial colloidal clearance function. Living
BCG and other mycobacterial entities have been shown to magnify the
ability of reticuloendothelial cells to clear colloidal particles from the
circulation. This has been shown as well for MER (80). The i.p. administration of 0.5 mg MER to young adult male albino mice was followed almost immediately by a steep short-term rise in the rate of clearance of colloidal carbon, before any increase occurred in the size or
weight of liver or spleen. An even higher peak of total as well as of
functional carbon clearance occurred very rapidly upon giving the animals
a second injection of MER, 29 days after the first. A second spontaneous
peak of increased clearing activity was seen approximately two weeks
after the second MER exposure.

The rapidity of increased reticuloendothelial activity following a first
and second injection of MER was perhaps somewhat greater than that
obtained by other workers with living BCG.

Mice treated first with MER and then, some weeks later, with other
substances capable of magnifying reticuloendothelial function also displayed an anamnestic peaking of clearance rates.

The time intervals between MER administration and tumor challenge
which were usually found optimal in other studies for a maximum MER
protective effect coincided, on the whole, with the period after treatment
at which carbon clearance rates had returned to normal, but still showed
a virtually instantaneous climb upon second stimulation. It would appear
reasonable to assume that implantation of tumor isografts and microbial
challenge by themselves constitute such a second RES stimulatory effect.
The time patterns of RES stimulation by MER may thus be causally
connected with those of MER-elicited nonspecific resistance. On the
other hand, not too much significance can be attached to the carbon
clearance data because it has been shown (81, 82) that there may be
little correlation between clearing activities vis-à-vis different colloids,

---

significantly increased the strength of the immune reaction of mice responding to
the development of implants of premalignant mammary tissue.

Bekesi (personal communication) has found that MER confers a marked
protection against the development of spontaneous and transplantable leukemias
in two inbred strains of mice.

or, for that matter, between the phagocytic capacities of reticuloendothelial cells in different organs.

Effects of MER on clearance of labeled antigen from the circulation and on its distribution in the body. Analysis of the effects of MER on the removal of antigenically active material from the blood stream and on its subsequent translocation, would contribute more to an understanding of the mechanisms of the nonspecific immunogenicity of MER than data coming from the colloidal carbon clearance experiments. Accordingly, a study has been initiated (83, 84) to follow the body distribution of i.p. injected, nonaggregated I^{125}-bovine γ-globulin (BGG). This substance is a very poor immunogen in mice, and frequently elicits a state of specific immunological unresponsiveness; MER-stimulated animals, in contrast, are able to produce antibodies to the protein (see below).

In the first hours after injection, as the antigen passes into the circulation from the peritoneal cavity, blood levels increased in all the mice, but always to a significantly lesser extent in MER-treated animals. During this early period, the liver, mesenteric lymph node, intestine and lungs of the treated mice concentrated more of the label, whereas the spleen levels were lower than in the controls. After several hours and up to one week later, however, all of these organs contained less antigen than those of the controls, and blood levels were similar. During the same period of time, the amounts of label in the urine and feces of MER-treated mice were considerably higher than in the excreta of the controls. These observations point to a more rapid degradation and elimination of the labeled antigen in the tissues of treated subjects, following a more effective early uptake by a number of organs.

Many investigators have suggested that, for an antigen to be effectively immunogenic, it should have ready access to immunologically reactive tissue, while unprocessed antigen should rapidly decrease to levels below the threshold of tolerigenicity. The results so far obtained from studies on the clearance and translocation of labeled BGG are thus compatible with the hypothesis that MER has a stimulatory effect on the immunogenic capacity of this antigen, and hence on immunological reactivity against it.

Effects of MER on lymphoid tissue morphology. Initial experiments on the effects of MER pretreatment on the IgM response of Swiss Webster albino and BALB/c mice to SRBC revealed a frequent increase in the size, weight and cellularity of the spleens of animals given one or two injections of 0.5 mg each of MER i.p., followed several days to two weeks later by immunization with SRBC by the same route (80). Spleen enlargement was generally greater and more consistent when two injections of MER were given. These studies also revealed a frequently more pronounced effect of MER on the appearance of specifically reactive plaque-forming (i.e., IgM-synthesizing) cells (PFC) in the spleens of the animals than on general cellularity, and the specific stimulation of cells producing antibodies to SRBC was seen even at times when there was no general increase in spleen weight or cellular content.

Subsequent studies (D. Yashphe and Y. Boss, in preparation) showed that i.p. injection of MER alone, without subsequent immunization, at times caused similar splenic enlargement. Spleen size and weight began to increase several days to a week after MER administration, and then increased progressively for some time, with ultimate weights reaching up to two to three times the normal value. Significant modifications of fine structure of the spleen were not, however, discernible after MER administration.

It thus appears that exposure to MER heightens lymphoid tissue responsiveness both specifically towards antigens administered after treatment, and broadly in terms of a general hyperplastic reaction. Furthermore, the latter is not a condition for the manifestation of the former.

In order to characterize better the general effects of MER on lymphoid tissue, the lymph nodes of mice draining the sites of MER application were compared histologically with distal lymphoid centers. In these experiments, MER was administered without any additional antigenic stimulation. Only preliminary results are so far available.

When MER was injected into the food pad of one hind leg, the size and weight of the draining popliteal lymph nodes increased up to six-fold within five days of administration. Contralateral popliteal nodes and peripheral lymph nodes exhibited no such change.

The popliteal nodes of normal mice generally show little histological evidence of immunological activity; they consist of a thin cortex and a loosely textured paracortical area. In contrast, the draining popliteal nodes of MER-treated animals showed considerable hyperplasia of the paracortical region, but with little additional follicle formation. Such an effect was not obvious in distal lymph nodes.

The histological picture of the draining popliteal nodes of MER-stimulated mice resembled that seen in nodes during the course of a cellular immune reaction (85; D. Yashphe and J. Boss, in preparation). The paracortical hyperplasia is due largely to thymus-derived lymphocytes T cells), the immunocytes which appear to play an auxiliary role in the production of antibodies to most antigens and which are held to be the effector cells in cellular immunity (86, 87). Whether the similar changes induced by MER reflect physiological effects on lymphoid tissue, nonspecific heightening of cellular immunological reactivity to incidental antigens, or the development of specific cellular hypersensitivity against some of the MER protein components, remains to be explored.

MER can heighten states of resistance and of immunological responsiveness in many systems even when it is administered by a different route than the eventual antigenic or parasitic challenge. The observations already made that MER alters the appearance of adjacent but not of distal lymphoid centers suggest that gross changes in lymphoid tissue at the portals of entry or lodgement of antigens, microorganisms, or tumor cells are not requisite for a manifestation of MER-induced heightened responsiveness. It is possible, instead, that more subtle, histologically undetectable changes do occur in distal lymphoid tissue following MER administration or, alternatively, that cells with altered reactivity migrate from activated sites in response to the challenge. It would thus appear that MER acts differently from certain other fractions of mycobacteria, for instance trehalose-6,6-dimycolate (cord factor), which prevent the development of carcinogen-induced neoplasms in target tissue where, and presumably because, the agent has initiated diffuse granuloma formation (88).

Effects of MER on macrophages. It is held by most immunologists today that at least some antigens must be "processed" by macrophagic cells before they can actually function as operative immunogens, or, alternatively, that removal of excess and potentially tolerigenic amounts of antigens must be effected by macrophages to permit an active immune response (89–91). Knowledge of the effects of MER on macrophage physiology might contribute, therefore, to our understanding of the substance's mode of nonspecific immunological activity, and studies have recently been initiated in our laboratories by Drs. Ruth Galily and Edith Wiener to determine the existence and nature of such effects.

In preliminary experiments, C3H mice were injected i.p. with 0.5 mg MER. One week later, cells were obtained from the animals by flushing their peritoneal cavities with saline. The macrophages were separated from the other peritoneal washing cells by permitting them to attach to the walls of Petri dishes for several hours, and their enzyme content was assayed (92). The results to date show a 20- to 100-fold increase in the levels of active acid phosphatase and cathepsin D over those seen in macrophages similarly obtained from saline-treated donors. It also appeared that contact with MER *in vitro* considerably heightens the cell content of acid phosphatase.

Although these findings are still only preliminary, they already suggest that MER has an effect on macrophage physiology. The increased enzymatic capacity of these cells may well represent a heightened ability to degrade ingested material, which, to begin with, may be phagocytized more effectively in MER-treated animals, and perhaps to render it more immunogenic by exposing reactive sites.

Effects of MER on humoral antibody formation and on the appearance of antibody-producing cells. 1) Responsiveness to a large particulate antigenic entity: heterogeneic and allogeneic red blood cells: Mice of several inbred strains (C3H, C3H/2, BALB/c and BALB/cfC3H) and outbred Swiss albino mice were employed in these studies (80, 93–95).

In young adult animals, treatment by one or two i.p. injections of 0.5 mg MER each, at a time ranging from several days to several months prior to immunization with SRBC or allogeneic (Strain A) red cells, usually accelerated the appearance of lymphoid cells producing both IgM and IgG antibodies, increased the maximum numbers of these cells totally (per spleen) and relatively (per unit number of nucleated spleen cells), accelerated and heightened the titers of circulating hemagglutinins and prolonged markedly high-level plateaus of both specifically reactive cells and antibody titers. Two pretreatments with MER were generally more effective than only one, and the usually optimum time schedule of MER administration was found to be 14 and 3 days preceding immunization. Other time intervals were often also highly effective, however, and in some instances single pretreatment elicited heightened responsiveness to a similar extent as dual administration.

In outbred albino mice 10 weeks of age or younger, however, pretreatment with MER either elicited no effect or, when administration was very shortly before immunization, significantly reduced the number of IgM-reactive lymphoid cells. Such a reduction was never seen in older outbred mice, nor in mice of the inbred strains even when these were only 8 to 10 weeks old at the time of MER exposure. This observation thus illustrates that not only the parameters of MER treatment and specific immunization, but also host genotype, can influence the outcome of the nonspecific stimulation.

The stimulatory action of MER pretreatment was most marked when antigenic stimulation was weak (with a small number of foreign red cells); with very large antigenic stimuli, leading by themselves to maximal antibody responses, only a small additional effect could usually be seen for MER pretreatment (96).

The very rapid emergence of reactive cells and release of antibodies in MER pretreated animals may be of more than merely quantitative significance for host defense mechanisms. The distribution of antibodies among the different immunoglobulin classes varies with time following sensitization; different biological properties have been ascribed to the several molecular species of immunoglobulins; and the early macroglobulin response may play a particularly important role in the destruction of foreign pathogenic cells (97–99). It has, indeed, been suggested that the early events following contact with a pathogen may be determinative of the final outcome of the interaction (100).

MER pretreatment appeared to be most effective in stimulating primary antibody responsiveness when specific immunization was by the same route (D. J. Yashphe, in preparation). (In many of the cellular immune responsiveness systems, however, and in many of the antimicrobial and antitumor resistance models, this is not a condition for efficacy.)

Administration of MER at the time of red blood cell immunization was also effective in many instances in heightening primary antibody formation. MER given after immunization with a high dose of SRBC when a primary response was already manifest, did not change the levels of PFC or hemagglutinin titers. When priming was with low doses of SRBC, treatment with MER initiated after the primary response was evident did elevate the levels of circulating antibodies (PFC numbers were not determined in these experiments).

These and other observations point to the likelihood that MER, and perhaps also other nonspecific stimulators of immunological reactivity, may act both in terms of the number of specifically reactive lymphoid cells and in terms of their capacity to synthesize and secrete free immunoglobulins with specific activity.

Decline in the number of primary IgM PFC in MER-pretreated mice was slow despite the appearance of large numbers of IgG antibody-producing cells, thus suggesting that small quantities of IgG might have less of a feedback inhibitory effect on IgM production in the treated than in normal hosts (D. J. Yashphe, in preparation).

In a further series of experiments, the effects of MER administration on the circulating antibody responses to a secondary SRBC immunization were analyzed. MER given before primary immunization, or between primary and secondary antigenic challenge, ultimately stimulated the magnitude and duration of the secondary response in most instances, but on occasion markedly reduced it in its early phases (94, 95). This delay in onset and peak development of secondary responsiveness was specific for the primary antigenic stimulus. Thus, mice immunized with SRBC and then treated twice with MER showed the same high primary and secondary reactivity to immunization with T2 phage as did animals pretreated with MER only (D. J. Yashphe, in preparation).

The secondary hemagglutinin response in normal mice was less than optimum when the animals were primed with high doses of SRBC. Pretreatment with MER prevented this inhibition, which has been likened to tolerance.

The delay in secondary responsiveness may also be of significance to the understanding of the mode of nonspecific protection elicited by MER against neoplastic cells: The secondary immune response is characterized by a predominance of IgG, rather than of IgM, antibodies, even shortly after its initiation. A retardation of the secondary response could thus be interpreted as a delay, perhaps crucial, in the peak production of those immune factors which can bring about the enhancement of foreign cells.

These observations suggest that MER enlarges the effective immunogenicity of SRBC, by potentiating the efficiency of antigen processing, or by increasing the sensitivity of antigen-sensitive cells, or by enlarging the number of these cells (95). Increasing the effective dose of antigen may, in turn, lead to decreased immunological memory (95, 96), either through a reduction in the pool of memory cells, or a lessened reactivity of memory cells to antigen, or a differentiation of at least some memory cells to cells poorly capable, though perhaps only temporarily, of active antibody production. Both the rapid stimulation of the primary response by MER pretreatment, and the slowing of the secondary response, followed by higher peaks and prolonged high levels of secondary reactivity, could thus be viewed within the framework of an MER-induced direction of the immune response away from memory and towards active antibody production.

2) Responsiveness to a small particulate antigenic entity: T2 bacteriophage: The consequences of MER treatment for production of antibody to T2 phage, and the parameters governing MER activity in this system were, on the whole, very similar to those seen vis-à-vis foreign red cells. The notable exception was that treatment with MER prior to first im-

munization, or between first and second antigenic exposure, did not bring about a delay in secondary responsiveness, but instead both accelerated and heightened it significantly (93–95; D. J. Yashphe, in preparation). Whether this difference in the effect of MER on the secondary reaction to SRBC and T2 phage is related to the difference in particle size of these two entities or to their distinctive chemical nature, remains to be ascertained.

3) Responsiveness to a soluble protein antigen—BGG: Experiments were performed (83, 84) with nonaggregated, soluble BGG, which is either only very weakly or not at all immunogenic for most mice, or in fact tolerigenic. The test animals, of the BALB/c strain, failed to give a primary antibody response to the protein, but were able to do so after exposure to MER. Treated young adults responded to dosages of BGG ranging from 100 μg to 10 mg BGG, antibody appearing in the circulation as early as seven days after immunization. Optimal MER stimulation was effected by two i.p. injections of 0.5 mg each, 14 and 3 days before antigen was given. A secondary response was elicited by alum-precipitated BGG in animals primed with the nonaggregated antigen (but not responding to it) and was elevated in those treated with MER prior to first immunization.

Mice given 0.1 mg MER i.p. already during the first week of life showed a strong primary response following BGG immunization at the age of five weeks, and both an accelerated and a heightened secondary reaction to alum-precipitated antigen administered four weeks after primary exposure. Similar observations were made in mice given MER and soluble BGG during the first and second weeks of life, respectively, and boosted with alum-precipitated protein four weeks later. The secondary antibody titers of control animals first immunized with soluble BGG in the second week of life (and which showed no primary response) were lower than in those first immunized at the age of five weeks (which also did not give a primary reaction), suggesting that a state of partial tolerance was induced in these mice by very early contact with the antigen. Pretreatment with MER in the first week after birth partly offset this development of tolerance.

MER appeared to be more strikingly effective in very young than in adult mice. For instance, primary anti-BGG activity was stimulated when the antigen was given even one month after MER treatment of neonates, whereas in young adults this long interval between MER and antigen administration was ineffective at a similar MER-body weight dose relationship.

These findings thus make two significant points: For one, MER pretreatment can render animals responsive to subsequently administered substances which are otherwise not actively immunogenic, in this case because of physical reasons (the soluble state of the heterologous protein); and MER pretreatment can prevent or break, at least to some extent, states of specific immunological unresponsiveness. These modulating capacities of MER could also be of direct significance to its mode of nonspecific protective action, because antigens of some microbial and neoplastic parasites may lack operative immunogenicity for physical or chemical reasons, or may be actively tolerigenic. The counteraction by MER of nonimmunogenicity and tolerigenicity thus complements its ability, described above, to further resistance rather than enhancement when administration is closely associated in time with specific antigenic stimulation. MER thus appears to emerge as an agent able to prevent, under some circumstances at least, various forms of immunological failure.*

In view of the fact that at least some infectious and many neoplastic diseases occur more frequently, and sometimes as more fulminating processes, in very young and very old individuals, that is, before and after the peak of immunological capacity is reached (101, 102), the relation between the effectiveness of MER immune stimulation and age in poorly reactive subjects is of special interest. Further comparative experiments showed that MER could strongly potentiate the circulating antibody response of immature inbred mice and retired breeders, in whom immunological capacity is less developed than in mature adults. Thus, the titers of antibodies to SRBC in four to seven-week-old and in 38-week-old BALB/c NIV females were brought to the level seen in normal 17- to 19-week-old animals by treatment with MER prior to immunization (D. J. Yashphe, in preparation); however, the antibody levels in the

---

* It is noted that some investigators today consider certain states of "specific immunological unresponsiveness," notably against foreign cells, which are induced by contact with antigen to be not *bona fide* unresponsiveness, but rather immunological enhancement due to antibody formation (103). The mechanisms by which MER prevents specific immunological unresponsiveness (or tolerance) could thus be diverse, involving in some circumstances a direction of the immune response towards elements which do not bring about enhancement, and in others a true substitution of some degree of reactivity for an antigen-facilitated clonal deletion or "turning off."

treated young and aged mice remained somewhat lower than those of the MER-treated mature adults.

The synthetic polynucleotide poly-A:U and bacterial endotoxin have also been shown capable of stimulating antibody formation to SRBC in otherwise nonresponding newborn mice (104, 105), but the effects of these materials appear to be short-lived (105).

Administration of normal isogenic adult macrophages also confers on neonatal mice the ability to respond to SRBC (106). The MER effect seen in the BGG system could thus be due to an activation, perhaps an accelerated maturation, of immunocompetent cells, or to an altered ability of macrophages to "process" crude antigens into effective immunogens, or to both. (It was noted in earlier studies in guinea pigs that administration of tubercle bacillus entities to fetuses *in utero* several weeks before birth does, in fact, hasten the maturation of lymphoid tissue).

4) Miscellaneous observations on the stimulating effects of MER on humoral antibody formation: In experiments performed by Dr. David Nelken of our Department involving the production in mules of antibodies to rat skin, it was noted that animals given two doses of 10 mg MER s.c., 14 and 3 days before specific immunization, had significantly higher circulating antibody titers than normal mules or those given the skin preparation together with Freund's complete adjuvant.

Preliminary findings in our laboratory with another antigen, keyhole limpet hemocyanin (KLH), also showed that treatment of mice with MER prior to first immunization can stimulate very markedly both primary and secondary antibody production, with quantities of the antigen ranging from 1 to 100 μg (R. Gallily and E. Wiener, in preparation).

Studies are now under way on the effects of MER vis-à-vis production of antibody to antigens, such as components of bacterial flagella, which do not, apparently, require the participation of T-cells in the circulating antibody response (see also below).

5) Appearance of rosette-forming cells (RFC): In both normal animals and animals immunized with foreign erythrocytes, lymphoid cells can be found which bind red cells to their surface in the form of "rosettes" (107). RFC against other antigens are also found, and their presence is revealed by the use of RBC coated with these antigens. RFC are also known as antigen-binding cells (ABC) or antigen-reactive cells (ARC). The number of RFC is much larger in an immunized than in a normal

animal. Few of these cells actively produce specific antibodies, and they can be separated from PFC experimentally (108).

Nonantibody-secreting RFC may be identical with the antigen-reactive cells whose specific receptor interaction with antigen triggers the series of processes which lead to active antibody formation. They are hetero-geneous and appear to consist of both thymus-derived (T) and bone marrow-derived (B) lymphocytes; the former may be helper cells or memory cells or both, and the latter may as well constitute precursors of antibody-producing cells (109, 110).

In experiments begun only recently, it was found that mice treated with MER and subsequently immunized with SRBC showed four to five times the number of nonantibody-producing RFC per spleen as immunized animals pretreated with saline only, and that the increased RFC levels were maintained for several weeks (74; C. Abraham and D. J. Yashphe, in preparation). It thus appears that MER may affect immunological responsiveness at a very early stage in the ontogeny of a given response, by increasing the numbers of ARC, as well as terminally by increasing the numbers of antibody-forming cells and by expediting antibody secre-tion.

In the mouse, the relative numbers of thymus- and bone marrow-derived RFC can be determined by use of antisera directed towards the θ antigen, which is located on the surface of thymus cells and thymus-derived lymphocytes (109, 111, 112). Experiments are now under way to determine the differential effect of MER on these cell types. It is already apparent that, at least under some circumstances, MER stimulates the appearance of both types of lymphoid cells.

6) General comments: MER is emerging from these studies as an effective stimulator of antibody formation in mice, and perhaps in other species as well, to antigens of diverse nature, and under a variety of experimental conditions. Within the dose limits effective in eliciting anti-microbial and antitumor protection, MER was never seen to depress anti-body reactivity of adult animals to the test antigens employed. MER also elevated the immunological ability of immature mice, with the one noted exception in the case of young outbred albino mice where reactivity to SRBC was depressed when immunization followed shortly after treatment. The effect of much larger doses of MER on the antibody response was not tested.

As has been discussed above, enhancement of certain tumors is some-times engendered by MER at dosages and under experimental conditions which lead to heightened resistance against other tumors. Immunological enhancement is mediated by circulating antibodies,* and different tumors evince different degrees of susceptibility to enhancement or destruction by the various classes of immunoglobulin. There is no contradiction, therefore, between a consistently positive effect of MER on antibody formation over a range of 0.1 to 1.0 mg and its variable effects on tumor resistance.

A parallel series of studies has been initiated in our laboratories to ascertain the effect of MER on cellular immune reactivity to defined antigenic entities. The findings coming from these experiments may prove to be of particular importance, not only in casting further light on the mechanisms of the protective effects ascribable to MER, but also in leading to the development of more pertinent tests for the early determination of the likely consequences of treatment for states of resistance in individual recipients. In host-parasite relationships, where a parallelism can be established between high levels of host resistance and the predominant type of immunological reactivity to antigens of the parasite, early information on the direction of the MER-induced immunological effects to these, and perhaps also to other, test antigens, may facilitate variation of the necessary treatment. In principle, this consideration applies as well to any other nonspecific or specific immunogenic stimulus.

Effects of MER on cellular immunological reactivity. 1) Response of inbred female mice to male skin isografts: A proportion of female mice reject second, and even first, male skin isografts, because of immune reactions mounted against antigen(s) controlled by the male Y chromosome. Sensitized lymphoid cells play the dominant role, and free antibodies at best an auxiliary one, in these rejections (114–116). Animals of immunologically competent strains show such reactivity more frequently than those of strains characterized by lower general immune capacity, and lines of mice have been ranked in terms of immunological strength by the criterion of female rejection of male grafts (117).

In a series of exploratory experiments, the effects of pretreatment with MER on the frequency of primary male skin isograft acceptance by female mice and on the length of survival of grafts eventually rejected

---

* The suggestion has recently been advanced that perhaps even sensitized lymphoid cells may, under special circumstances, evoke enhancement rather than heightened tumor resistance (113). The value of these cells to hosts faced with the challenge of neoplasia may thus not be as decisively unambiguous as has been commonly accepted.

were assessed (118). One or two injections of 0.5 mg MER administered i.p. several days or weeks before skin transplant challenge did not increase the already high incidence of rejection by C57Bl females, nor was there persuasive evidence of a shortened lifespan of the grafts. In contrast, MER did bring about a heightened incidence of graft rejection in females of the C3H genotype, in whom the frequency of rejection is low; the longevity of the ultimately rejected grafts was shortened.

A major disadvantage of skin-graft rejection as a criterion of cellular immunological responsiveness is the difficulty of quantitating the kinetics and extent of the attack on the target tissue. We therefore chose two models of cellular reactivity which lend themselves better to quantification and which are described in the following sections.

2) Response of C57Bl and C3Hf mice to allografts of a BALB/c plasma cell tumor (PCT): C3Hf and C57Bl male mice were given one or two consecutive injections of 0.5 mg MER i.p., 3 to 30 days prior to administration by the same route of 0.5 to 5.0 $\times$ 10^7 living cells of a PCT originating in a BALB/c male repeatedly injected with mineral oil (119, 120). The PCT allograft never grew progressively. Ten days after allograft immunization, the recipients were sacrificed and separate cell suspensions prepared of their spleens, mesenteric lymph nodes and pooled distal lymph nodes. The ability of the lymphoid cells to attack PCT target cells was assayed *in vitro,* employing the technique of Brunner et al. (121) in which target cell damage is assessed by the liberation of labeled chromium (Cr^{51}) from cell constituents. The amounts of Cr^{51} released from the target cells in contact with varying numbers of immune lymphoid cells derived from donors pretreated with MER or with saline (the controls included in each experiment) were compared with those released from target cells incubated with similar numbers of lymphoid cells from normal mice. The differences in the values represent the release of Cr specifically elicited by the immune effector cells, and directly indicate the extent of cell injury.

In over 30 such experiments, the cell damage caused by immune lymphoid cells from MER-pretreated mice was consistently and significantly greater than that caused by lymphoid cells from nontreated animals (122). The MER effect was evident in terms of greater Cr release at similar effector cell/target-cell ratios, and also in terms of the numbers of effector cells required to release a given quantity of the label in a given period of time. Lymphoid cells from the local and distal nodes as well as from the spleen were active.

Spleen cells taken from MER-treated but nonimmunized animals and injected into irradiated isogenic hosts subsequently exposed to the PCT allograft, transferred the MER-heightened lymphoid cytotoxic efficacy to the recipients (123). The amount of raw MER which could conceivably have been transferred in this procedure from the treated donors to the recipients would be much too small to evoke a primary effect in the latter. It appears, therefore, that the MER effect on cellular immunity resides, at least as a terminal manifestation, in the spleen cell population employed in the passive transfer.

In this model, the fact that the target cells are neoplastic is obscured by the fact that they are allogeneic, i.e., the immune response to them is directed largely or solely against the histocompatibility antigens which distinguish BALB/c from C3H and C57Bl tissues. In addition, MER was also effective in increasing lymphoid cell cytotoxic potency in an isogenic system, in which the response of BALB/c animals to the same PCT was measured (123); the tumor was previously shown to have a low level of tumor-associated antigenicity (120).

Soluble mediators of cell damage did not appear to be responsible for the liberation of Cr in this test system, and it seems that the cytotoxic effect of the immune lymphoid cells is here caused in large part by direct cell-to-cell interaction.

Release of Cr from target cells, as well as loss of the ability to exclude certain dyes, are indications of relatively severe damage. In order to assess earlier and less acute cytotoxic effects, more sensitive criteria were recently developed by Mr. Michael Steinitz and Mr. Zami Ben Sasson of our laboratory. These are based on changes in the facility of target cells to synthesize protein, RNA and DNA as indicated by a depressed incorporation of labeled precursors into these macromolecules. These changes are manifested very soon after contact with sensitized effector cells and before the occurrence of detectable dye uptake or Cr release (124), and preliminary observations suggest that MER heightens the ability of immune lymphocytes to trigger these early metabolic disturbances.

3) Response of guinea pigs to immunization with protein-hapten conjugates which are by themselves very poorly immunogenic: In a series of experiments conducted together with Dr. S. Ben-Efraim of Tel Aviv University (122), outbred albino guinea pigs were treated with various quantities of MER (1.0 to 5.0 mg) administered by different routes (i.p., s.c., i.c. and into the footpads) either 7 or 14 days before chal-

lenge with antigen or simultaneously with the antigen. The MER was suspended in saline or in incomplete Freund's adjuvant (IFA). The antigen was a dinitrophenyl-guinea pig globulin conjugate (DNP-GPG), containing nine moles DNP/mole protein, which does not by itself elicit an immune response in guinea pigs, but does so when incorporated in Freund's adjuvant. Sensitization with the antigen was by injection into all four footpads of a total of 10 μg, given in saline, IFA, or complete Freund's adjuvant (CFA). The animals were tested for skin hypersensitivity reaction to DNP-GPG one, two and three weeks later, and for the presence of serum antibodies against the conjugate by Boyden's indirect hemagglutination test (125).

All hypersensitivity reactions were of typical delayed type. As expected, administration of the conjugate together with CFA resulted in the development of both delayed hypersensitivity (DH) and humoral antibody formation; administration in IFA also facilitated antibody formation, but none of these animals exhibited DH. CFA introduced alone at the same site, seven days before sensitization, was effective in permitting development of DH in some of the guinea pigs, but not antibody formation. When the interval between the injection of CFA and antigen was 14 days, neither type of response was seen. Similarly, CFA given i.p. prior to sensitization was ineffective. In contrast, i.p., s.c. or i.c. administration of MER in saline one or two weeks before sensitization led to DH responses in a large number of animals, but to humoral antibody formation in only a few. When MER was suspended in IFA, however, pretreatment failed to evoke DH, but did permit antibody formation in some instances. Application of the conjugate together with MER in an aqueous vehicle led to neither DH nor antibody response, but substitution of whole tubercle bacilli by MER in CFA given together with the conjugate facilitated the development of both types of reaction.

MER can thus take the place of whole tubercle bacilli in a conventional adjuvant situation, not surprising in view of the fact that MER is a crude fraction of the organisms. It is also evident, however, that MER is capable of preparing the animals to respond to the conjugate with DH under circumstances in which CFA is totally ineffective, that is, when treatment is removed in time and place from sensitization. In order to be effective as pretreatment, MER had to be presented in a "free" form, not in admixture with IFA. MER thus emerges as an agent able to affect the immunological apparatus in a manner which quantitatively or qualitatively goes beyond the classical adjuvant effect of water-in-oil emulsions containing whole tubercle bacilli.

Furthermore, depending on the circumstances of administration, MER often preferentially stimulates either DH or antibody formation, but usually not both types of response simultaneously. This is also apparent from further experiments, in which sensitization was with a stronger antigen, the conjugate of DNP with a heterologous protein, human serum albumin (HSA). MER pretreatment of an animal challenged with 10 μg DNP-HSA distinctly favored antibody formation. However, when the amount of antigen was reduced to 1 μg, antibody formation did not occur, but DH was again elicited.

These observations may be consistent with the view of some immunologists that DH reactions precede the production of free antibodies in a given immune response, and that DH represents the response to a minimal antigenic stimulus. Thus, the development of MER pretreatment may succeed in permitting an animal to mount DH to a sensitization which would otherwise be entirely ineffective, but may not be able to direct the response further. In contrast, when MER functions as a classical, strong adjuvant, replacing tubercle bacilli in CFA administered together with the antigen, the stimulation may be sufficient to elicit a full-fledged immunological reaction. It is also possible that once circulating antibody production is stimulated in this system, DH is depressed by antibody-mediated feedback mechanisms. This possibility is currently under investigation.

In any event, the findings suggest that MER pretreatment may selectively favor cellular or humoral responsiveness to an antigen, depending on the conditions of treatment and the strength of the immunogenic stimulus. Tumor-associated antigens are generally considered to be relatively weak immunogens, at least in the autochthonous and isogenic host. The possibility of modulating the immune response against them in the direction of cellular immunity, by appropriate manipulation of the parameters of MER administration and tumor antigen immunization or hyperimmunization, may accordingly be the most exciting implication of these observations.

4) General comments: It is apparent from these studies on the effects of MER on cellular immunity that the agent can act on immunologically reactive tissue before contact with antigen, altering the tissue's subsequent ability to respond to such contact. In some systems at least, a latent period before antigenic challenge is required for the manifestation of MER

efficacy. A rapid distribution of MER in the tissues may be required, as suggested by the failure of the substance to act when it was incorporated in IFA and employed as pretreatment in guinea pigs then immunized with protein-hapten conjugates. It is thus not inconceivable that very small but critical amounts of MER, perhaps after having undergone marked alterations by processing macrophages, may have to reach lymphoid or reticuloendothelial tissue distal from the point of administration. A similar requirement may explain the greater effectiveness of MER pretreatment in some humoral antibody formation models when it is given by the same route as the antigen.

The ability of MER to stimulate antibody production and resistance to microbial pathogens and neoplastic cells can also be initiated before exposure to the antigen or parasite. Although a latent period is not always required in the antibody and resistance systems, the effects of pretreatment are commonly more striking than those of treatment immediately before or after challenge.

It also appears that cellular and humoral reactivity may be stimulated to different extents, even towards the same antigen, under different conditions of MER pretreatment, and that marked stimulation of the one may go hand in hand with lack of effect on the other. It may therefore be possible to define, at least empirically, the parameters of MER nonspecific stimulation and of specific immunization which will favor given forms of responsiveness to given antigens and pathogenetic cells.

Effects of MER on immunological responsiveness of animals exposed to whole body irradiation and to treatment with antilymphocytic (ALS) and antithymocytic (ATS) sera and cortisone. The observations that treatment with MER can stimulate immunological reactivity in natively deficient animals, and that it can evoke heightened tumor resistance in mice given chemotherapy with immunosuppresive agents, suggested further exploration of the possible capability of MER to reverse states of induced immunosuppression. Initial experiments have been conducted with whole-body irradiation and with exposure to ALS, ATS and cortisone.

Studies of the immunostimulatory effects of MER in irradiated mice are still in progress. It is already apparent, however, that the immune reactivity to one test antigenic material, SRBC, in BALB/c mice first irradiated with 400 or 550 R, treated i.p. 1 and again 11 days later with 0.5 mg MER and immunized three days thereafter, is not improved in comparison with that of saline-injected. irradiated hosts, but is actually depressed. In contrast, MER treatment given prior to irradiation offered some protection against the radiation-induced immunosuppression (126).

Further experiments with animals of other strains and species, and with different dosages and timing of irradiation and MER treatment, are under way. The findings so far suggest that treatment begun after extensive destruction of immunologically reactive tissue has taken place may in fact be futile, or that the reviving immune capacity in such subjects may be "preempted" (127, 128) by the subsequent contact with MER, itself an antigenic entity. In current experiments, emphasis is therefore being placed on the suggested protective effects of MER applied prior to irradiation.

In experiments in which immunosuppression was effected by means of ATS, MER largely reversed the depressed ability to respond to SRBC under similar experimental circumstances, when treatment was initiated both before and after administration of the serum.

ALS was studied in a cellular immunity system, the *in vitro* cytotoxic action of C57Bl and C3Hf immune lymphocytes against BALB/c PCT target cells. Under circumstances in which the administration of ALS completely abolished the specific cytotoxic activity of the animals' spleen cells, the lymphoid cells of immunized mice treated with 0.5 mg MER several days preceding exposure to the serum remained as effective as those from immunized animals not exposed to ALS and stimulated with MER (74, 123).

The influence of MER on immunological reactivity depressed by cortisone is being investigated in mice using a SRBC-RFC model. Cortisone (125 mg/kg body wt), administered two days after SRBC immunization, markedly lowered the number of RFC which appeared, most of the depressing effect being manifested against T-cells. Treatment of the animals with MER several days before immunization partly prevented the cortisone effect.

These observations, preliminary as they are, suggest that MER is capable of elevating and restoring a wide range of immunological functions, which extend to states of deficiency induced by at least some extrinsic agents.

DISCUSSION

Relationship of MER to other agents which have a nonspecific effect on immunological responsiveness and resistance states; terminology. Numerous substances, both of microbial and nonmicrobial origin, are capable of altering the immune response to other, antigenically unrelated entities (30, 31). Some of these agents have also been shown to raise or lower the resistance of higher animals to infectious microorganisms or malignant cells, or both, depending on the circumstances of treatment and challenge. In some instances, lowering and raising of resistance occur sequentially, especially in the case of gram-negative bacterial endotoxins (129). However, changes in immunological reactivity to defined antigens have not always been seen to go hand in hand with changes in states of resistance; some agents with confirmed high activity in one respect have so far exhibited only limited, or no, potency in the other. In some instances, the nonspecifically active substance must be given together with the antigen or pathogen (20, 73, 130), whereas in others, administration may be removed in time and place.

The nonspecific effects on immunological responsiveness to known antigens which are exerted by such substances are manifested in several major directions: quantitative increases in antibody titers or in the degree of cellular reactivity or both; changes in the distribution of antibodies between the different immunoglobulin classes and orientation of the response away from antibody production and towards cellular immunity; and a positive response towards antigens which lack sufficient immunogenicity and tend instead to lead to the development of specific unresponsiveness. It has been suggested that the terms "adjuvant" and "adjuvanticity" be employed to differentiate between some of these properties. Thus, Dresser proposes that "A 'conventional adjuvant' can be defined as a substance which increases the antibody titer to an immunogenic antigen. In contrast 'adjuvanticity' ... has a more restricted meaning, being the property of an antigen itself (intrinsic adjuvanticity) or a substance other than an antigen (extrinsic adjuvanticity) which leads an antigen to induce immunity rather than immunological paralysis" (131). Since such "conventional adjuvants" as Freund's adjuvant also prominently heighten cellular immunity and often preferentially stimulate its development, and since they can affect antibody distribution among the several molecular species of immunoglobulins, these properties are generally also subsumed under the term adjuvant.

It must be noted at once, however, that casual use of the terms "adjuvant" and "adjuvanticity" is likely to be misleading. The mechanisms which underlie "adjuvant" and "adjuvanticity" action remain obscure, and some agents can induce more than one effect, albeit under different conditions. In most instances, causal associations have not yet been established between the capacity of a substance to act as a conventional adjuvant or adjuvanticity agent and to alter states of resistance. Moreover, certain semantic implications attach to the term "adjuvant," and especially to adjuvants containing tubercle bacillus entities, despite evidence to the contrary. Thus, the mechanism of depot effect and a uniformly stimulatory result on immunological reactivity are often still automatically associated with Freund's and other adjuvants, despite persuasive information that "adjuvants activate lymphoid cells to an extent that cannot be explained simply by their role as an antigen depot" (130), and that pretreatment with some adjuvants, including Freund's, sometimes even depresses immunological reactivity (132–134). Conversely, the term adjuvant is not always read to encompass modifications of resistance as well as influences on defined immunological reactions.

It is suggested, therefore, that a broader and more inclusive term, "modulator," be substituted for adjuvant and adjuvanticity. This term has not been commonly used in the past to describe the heterogeneous and mechanistically ill-defined phenomena of nonspecifically directed variations in immunological responsiveness and resistance, and is thus relatively free of implicit connotations which may be erroneously restrictive. "Modulator" and "modulation" describe nonspecific properties and effects without any implied bias as to mode of action, and until precise mechanisms can be associated with distinct results, the terms can be used more safely and correctly to subsume the different manifestations of nonspecific effects on immunity.

As would be expected, MER shares behavioral properties with other nonspecific immunological modulators, and especially with other tubercle bacillus entities. It also clearly differs from other such agents in a number of crucial effects. Prominent among these are the long duration of its protective and immunostimulatory action when it is given before challenge, and even by a different route, and its very broad and often very considerable efficacy in inhibiting the development of neoplastic processes.

Although the active principle(s) of MER may fall within the family of lipopolysaccharide-protein macromolecular complexes, MER obviously does not behave like the gram-negative bacterial endotoxin LPS: It is not pyrogenic; it lacks the broadly toxic properties of LPS; its spectrum of resistance-stimulating activities is very different; and it does not cause negative phases of resistance to microbial pathogens prior to a period of elevated resistance.

Mode of MER action. The primary loci of MER action on the immunological apparatus are still unknown, but it is clear that its effects are ultimately expressed in terms of elevated RES function, heightened antibody-producing capacity of lymphoid tissue and increased cytotoxic potency of lymphoid effector cells. The conditions under which MER elevates immunological reactivity and corrects native and induced immunological deficiency are generally very similar to those which govern its success in magnifying refractoriness to microbial and neoplastic challenge. This strongly suggests (but does not yet prove) that the increased resistance bestowed by MER is indeed based on modulation of specific immunological ability.

The effects of MER on antibody formation appear to be manifested at several loci: by enlargement of the number of ARC in lymphoid tissue, and perhaps also by increase of their sensitivity to stimuli which direct their physiological maturation towards the capacity for antibody production; by changes in the number of memory cells or their receptivity to antigen-facilitated activation, or both; and directly by increase in the populations, and conceivably the persistence and efficiency, of cells' actively producing antibodies.

The effect on the numbers of antigen-sensitive cells is evident from the observations that MER pretreatment significantly raises RFC counts in the spleens of SRBC-immunized mice (C. Abraham and D. J. Yashphe, in preparation). Whether the subsequent immunological behavior of these same cells is also altered is not yet known.

Changes in the population of memory cells are suggested by the finding that the secondary antibody response is (ultimately) elevated in primed mice pretreated with MER (94, 95). The development of higher secondary peak titers of treated animals is, however, preceded in some systems by a delayed onset of the secondary response. This may reflect an initial reduction in the pool of memory cells, brought about by an induced maturation to active immunoglobulin-producing cells under the influence of MER, followed by overcompensation of the rapidity or efficiency with which the remaining memory and antigen-sensitive cells convert mature, antibody-producing cells. Alternatively, equal numbers of memory cells may remain in primed, MER-stimulated mice after the initial antibody response, but they may be transitorily less ready to move in the direction of active antibody formation.

The influence of MER on actively antibody-producing cells is compatible with several other observations: The agent is able to stimulate an ongoing primary antibody response to some antigens (94, 95); high primary and secondary titers are maintained longer, sometimes appreciably so, in treated animals (94–96); treatment permits mice to react with a strong primary response to nonaggregated BGG which, in normal animals, elicits a secondary response but fails to evoke an active primary one (84). Although the activity of MER is thus expressed in terms of changes in both the memory and the active antibody-producing compartments of immunological reactivity, it is not impossible that the primary locus of MER efficacy is on the level of antigen-sensitive cells. The other manifestations could conceivably reflect the consequences of effects on antigen-sensitive cells as shifts in the equilibrium of the functionally distinct units in the spectrum leading from antigen sensitivity to antibody production.

MER potentiates the function of T-cells, as is suggested by its stimulation of lymphoid cell cytotoxic capacity and perhaps also by its reversion, at least in part, of immunosuppression elicited by ATS. The latter effect could, however, arise from a compensatory enlargement of the immunological function of B-cells. Extensive experiments are now under way to define more precisely and in quantitative terms the effects of MER on T and B lymphoid cells.

Possible role of nonspecific modulators of resistance and immunological functions in nature. The extent of the distribution of nonspecifically active microbial moieties in nature is not known, and no attempt has been initiated to search for such agents systematically. It does appear, however, that such substances are strongly represented among several groups of bacteria which are ubiquitous in the environments of most higher animals, and many of which cause disease. These are the mycobacteria, corynebacteria, hemophilus and gram-negative bacilli.

There would be obvious survival value to the development of means by which exposure to such microorganisms is translated into broadly directed heightened resistance to superinfection. Recovery from debilitating microbial disease may indeed be difficult in the face of likely secondary infections, unless the preceding microbial contact leads to an umbrella of nonspecific protection, at least temporarily. It may well be that adaptation to exploit microbial contact in this direction represents a major phylogenetic basis for the phenomenon of microbially induced nonspecific resistance. However, even more fundamental physiological processes may depend on the nonspecific modulation of antigen-antibody interactions by microbial fractions. Two areas of such effects can be envisaged.

For one, many autochthonous body constituents are actively or at least potentially antigenic even when they are normal, and in all probability more pronouncedly so when they undergo the alterations of aging and become effete, when they are damaged by other circumstances, and when they undergo neoplastic transformations. It is an obvious condition of existence that autochtonous antigens do not commonly muster strong immune responses, but it may be equally essential that at times some degree of immunological reactivity develops toward them. Only a few such circumstances need be mentioned to make this point: Immunological recognition and reaction may be a vital component of the surveillance mechanism against cancer. Tolerance of self may not, in fact, be due to the absence of antiself reactive clones, but rather to the continuous production of enhancing antibodies (103). Recognition and disposal of worn-out and damaged tissues may be triggered by immunological reactions. The normal course of blastocyst implantation and of birth may involve immunological processes (135), and there is some reason to think that immunological reactions play a role in the equilibria of differentiation and dedifferentiation (136); it is not inconceivable that the limitation of tissue and organ volumes and boundaries is directed in part by immunological factors. It is also possible that antibodies are produced against mutant clones of lymphoid cells with receptors and making antibodies against self antigens or against exotic (and perhaps actually nonexistent) chemical determinants which never come into the experience of the animal. Such anti-antibody (idiotype) responses (137) of the autochthonous host may limit the number of "nonsense" antibodies produced, and may serve as a secondary control mechanism for the prevention of autoimmune pathologies.

The common denominator in all of these postulated circumstances is the weak immunogenicity of the antigens, and the likely requirement of magnification and modulation. Thus, for example, immunological surveillance against neoplastic cells may depend on fine adjustment of the response in the direction of cellular elements and of antibodies having cytotoxic and antienhancement ["unblocking" (138)] activity. Microbial modulators may play an essential role in such magnification and adjustment.

The second possible area of nonspecific immunological modulation which may be necessary for normal physiological functioning, lies with the response to extrinsic antigens. Contact with small quantities of a large variety of antigens is continuous. The immunological disposal of these antigens, some of which may be injurious even in relatively small amounts, may require magnification of responsiveness by microbial modulators. Another possible function may be imagined; although entirely speculative, it does not appear to be wholly far-fetched: Ongoing antibody-antigen interaction in the tissues and body fluids must cause a continuous, though very low, release of a variety of pharmacological mediators, such as histamine, from mast cells, platelets and other specialized cells. For some of these mediators, which are very widely distributed in the animal kingdom, convincing natural functions have not yet been proposed. Could it be, as others have suggested, that the normal tone of blood vessels and of smooth muscle is a manifestation of the ongoing release of such mediators, under the influence of low level antigen-antibody interactions, stimulated, in turn, by microbial modulators?

Some microbial and some nonmicrobial nonspecific immunological modulators may converge in terms of the molecular entities in which activity ultimately resides. It has been suggested, for instance, that nonspecifically active microbial moieties can also evoke specific hypersensitivity reactions; that the cell destruction brought about by these reactions leads to the accumulation of nucleic acid breakdown products; and that it is such substances which, like synthetic polynucleotides, produce the nonspecific changes in immunological competence (139, 140).

Concluding comments. MER has been discussed in this communication as a model of a broad category of substances which must be considered as frequently essential, nonspecific participants in the interaction of antigens with immunologically reactive tissue, both in nature and in experimental systems. MER has been shown capable of exerting profound effects on immunological function in a number of directions, and widely on resistance to microbial pathogens and neoplastic cells. Other nonspecific modulators of immunity undoubtedly also possess multifaceted potentials, and there is no reason to believe that the MER fraction represents the most effective or otherwise most desirable agent for nonspecific evocation of heightened resistance or orientation of immunological reactivity in wanted directions. At present, however, the high degree and wide range of efficacy which it displays, its safety and its stability make MER one of the most attractive available agents of nonspecific immunological modulation and potentiation of resistance.

The fact that MER is a crude, uncharacterized substance constitutes the major difficulty in further attempts to elucidate its mode of action and complicates its clinical exploitation. Nonetheless, MER is a consistently active and safe material despite this drawback, and it appears justified to have subjected it to broad biological study before initiating the difficult and uncertain effort of its purification and the identification of the active components. The advantages which would accrue from the availability of a purified, defined entity make this effort requisite, and work in this direction has been initiated (M. Tishler, in preparation). The mental reservation must be retained, however, that activity may ultimately come to be seen as residing in the physiochemical and biochemical properties of a mixture of macromolecular constituents, no one of which is potent by itself.

The work on MER described in this communication has been funded by research grants and contracts from a number of organizations and foundations, as well as by private supporters. This support is acknowledged with gratitude.

The major contributing organizations and foundations are the following: American Cancer Society; British Medical Research Council; The Cancer Research Fund, Chicago; Damon Runyon Memorial Fund for Cancer Research Inc.; Herbert A. Gorney Cancer Research Foundation; Ann Langer Memorial for Cancer Research; Samuel Lautenberg Memorial Fellowship; Leukemia Research Foundation Inc.; Carl Howard Litvin Fellowship Fund; National Institutes of Health (United States Public Health Service); Howard Netzky Memorial for Cancer Research; New York Cancer Research Institute; Rabbi Shai Shacknai Memorial Research Fund; Celia Sievitz Memorial Fellowship; West Coast Physicians Division of the American Friends of the Hebrew University.

Much of the more recent work on MER has been made possible by the support of Concern Foundation of Los Angeles, in memory of Beverly Wolman.

We express our special thanks and admiration for the generosity and large personal efforts on behalf of this work by Mr. and Mrs. Frank Lautenberg, Mr. and Mrs. Laurence A. Tisch, Mr. and Mrs. Henry Taub, Mr. and Mrs. Joseph Taub, Dr. and Mrs. Wilbur Schwartz.

It is not possible to cite individually all the many other individuals whose financial and personal commitments have furthered these studies and to whom we owe a debt of gratitude. We mention here only a few of those supporters and their families whose aid has been especially significant in permitting us to establish new programs of work in Jerusalem: Morris Bergreen, Robert Bernhard, Stanley Bogen, Ronald Cohen, Willard Chotiner, Wilbur Cowett, Paul Densen, Lester Finkelstein, the family and friends of the late Elaine Friedman, Maurice Goldblatt, Harry Goldman, Joseph Gottlieb and Abraham and Company, Albert Grosser, William Gumpert, Eliot Handler, friends of J. Ira Harris, Warren Hellman, Dr. Francis Hillman, Alfred Kleinbaum, George Kofman, Charles Krown, George Kramer, Arthur Kranseler, H.C. Krueger, friends of Frank Lautenberg, A. Lazaroff, Robert Litvin, Mrs. Roy Markus, Mrs. Eugenia Merwald, Paul Milstein, Seymour Milstein, Roy Neuberger, Jay Perry, Harold Price, Frederick Rose, Samuel Rothberg, Miles Rubin, Salomon Brothers, S. Scheuer, Melvin Seiden, Louis Sharpe, Barnett Shine, the Cancer Research Fund in memory of Violet Soll, Mickey

Spitalny, Bernard Stein, Herbert Stein, the Tibbians, friends of Laurence A. Tisch, the late Percy Uris, Clarence Unterberg, Lawrence Weinberg, in memory of the late Mata Weissman, Lewis Zorn. We also express our warm thanks to Mrs. Judith Weiss for her help with this manuscript.

REFERENCES

1. WILSON GS. The value of BCG vaccination in control of tuberculosis. *Br Med J* **2**: 855–859, 1947.
2. MYERS JA. A summary of the views opposing BCG. *Adv Tuberc Res* **8**: 272–303, 1957.
3. WEISS DW. Vaccination against tuberculosis with nonliving vaccines. I. The problem and its historical background. *Am Rev Resp Dis* **80**: 340–358, 495–509 and 676–688, 1959.
4. MIDDLEBROOK G. The mycobacteria, in: Dubos RJ and Hirsch JG (Eds), "Bacterial and mycotic infections of man," 4th edn. Philadelphia, JB Lippincott, 1965, p 490–529.
5. DUBOS RJ, SCHAEFER WB and PIERCE CH. Antituberculous immunity in mice vaccinated with killed tubercle bacilli. *J Exp Med* **97**: 221–233, 1953.
6. PEARSON L and GILLILAND SR. Some experiments upon the immunization of cattle against tuberculosis. *Phila Med J* **10**: 842, 1902.
7. LONG ER. Experimental infection-immunization against tuberculosis. *Arch Pathol Lab Med* **1**: 918–953, 1926.
8. GAISFORD W. The protection of infants against tuberculosis. *Br Med J* **2**: 1101–1106, 1955.
9. NEGRE L. Résistance antituberculeuse sans allergie conférée aux animaux de laboratoire par l'antigène méthylique. Etude de sa durée et de l'action préventive de ce produit associé à celle du BCG. *Ann Inst Pasteur (Paris)* **83**: 429–436, 1952.
10. WEISS DW and DUBOS RJ. Antituberculous immunity induced in mice by vaccination with killed tubercle bacilli or with a soluble bacillary extract. *J Exp Med* **101**: 313–330, 1955.
11. WEISS, DW and DUBOS R J. Antituberculous immunity induced by methanol extracts of tubercle bacilli—its enhancement by adjuvants. *J Exp Med* **103**: 73–85, 1956.
12. WEISS DW. Antituberculosis vaccination with non-living vaccines. *Tuberculology* **17**: 63–67, 1958.
13. WEISS DW. Antituberculosis vaccination in the guinea pig with non-living vaccines. *Am Rev Tuberc Pulm Dis* **77**: 719–724, 1958.
14. WILLIAMS CA and DUBOS RJ. Studies on fractions of methanol extracts of tubercle bacilli. I. Fractions which increase resistance to infection. *J Exp Med* **110**: 981–1004, 1959.
15. ESBER HJ, MENNINGER FF JR, TAYLOR DJ and BOGDEN AE. Methanol soluble fraction of *Mycobacterium butyricum*. Enhancement of the immune response in rats. *Cancer Res* (in press).
16. ESBER HJ, MENNINGER FF JR, TAYLOR DJ and BODGEN AE. Non-specific stimulation of tumor-associated immunity by methanol-soluble fraction of *Mycobacterium butyricum*. *Cancer Res* **32**: 795–803, 1972.
17. BILLINGHAM RE, BRENT L and MEDAWAR PB. "Actively acquired tolerance" of foreign cells. *Nature (Lond)* **172**: 603–606, 1953.
18. WEISS DW and WELLS AQ. Actively acquired tolerance to tuberculoprotein. *Nature (Lond)* **179**: 968–969, 1957.
19. WEISS DW. Inhibition of tuberculin skin hypersensitivity in guinea pigs by the injection of tuberculin and intact tubercle bacilli during fetal life. *J Exp Med* **108**: 83–104, 1958.

20. FREUND J. The mode of action of immunological adjuvants. *Adv Tuberc Res* **7** 130–148, 1956.
21. WEISS DW and MAIN O. The effect of pre- and neo-natally injected diphtheria toxoid on the homologous responsiveness of young guinea pigs—a preliminary report. *Immunology* **5**: 333–339, 1962.
22. SMITH RT. Immunological tolerance of nonliving antigens. *Adv Immunol* **1**: 67–129, 1961.
23. WEISS DW and WELLS AQ. Vaccination against tuberculosis with nonliving vaccines. II. Vaccination of guinea pigs with phenol-killed tubercle bacilli. *Am Rev Resp Dis* **81**: 518–538, 1960.
24. WEISS DW and WELLS AQ. Vaccination against tuberculosis with nonliving vaccines. III. Vaccination of guinea pigs with fractions of phenol-killed tubercle bacilli. *Am Rev Resp Dis* **82**: 339–357, 1960.
25. WESTPHAL O, NOWOTNY A, LUDERITZ O, HURNI H, EICHENBERGER E and SCHONHOLZER G. Die Bedeutung der Lipoid-Komponente (Lipoid A) für die biologischen Wirkungen bakterieller Endotoxine (Lipopolysaccharide). *Pharm Acta Helv* **33**: 401–411, 1958.
26. LANDY M, JOHNSON AG and GAINES S. Enhancement of antibody response to protein antigens by a lipopolysaccharide (endotoxin) derived from *Salmonella typhosa*. *Fed Proc* **13**: 499, 1954.
27. DUBOS RJ, WEISS DW and SCHAEDLER RW. Enhancing effect of adjuvants on the antituberculous immunity elicited in mice by methanol extracts of tubercle bacilli. *Am Rev Tuberc Pulm Dis* **75**: 781–784, 1956.
28. DUBOS RJ and SCHAEDLER RW. Reversible changes in the susceptibility of mice to bacterial infections. I. Changes brought about by injection of pertussis vaccine or of bacterial endotoxins. *J Exp Med* **104**: 53–65, 1956.
29. KIND LS. The altered reactivity of mice after inoculation with *Bordetella pertussis* vaccine. *Bacteriol Rev* **22**: 173–182, 1958.
30. SHILO M. Nonspecific resistance to infections. *Ann Rev Microbiol* **13**: 255–278, 1959.
31. YASHPHE DJ. Immunological factors in nonspecific stimulation of host resistance to syngeneic tumors. A review, in: Weiss, DW (Ed), "Immunological parameters of host-tumor relationships." New York, Academic Press, 1971, pp 90–107.
32. Beneficial effects of acute concurrent bacterial infections or toxin therapy on conditions other than cancer. New York, New York Cancer Research Institue, Inc, 1967.
33. NAUTS HC. The apparently beneficial effects of bacterial infections on host resistance to cancer. New York, New York Cancer Research Institute, 1969, Monograph 8.
34. BULLOCH W. "The history of bacteriology." London, Oxford University Press, 1960, pp 53–54.
35. BULLOCH W. "The history of bacteriology." London, Oxford University Press, 1960, pp 156–158.
36. BRETONNEAU P. Notice sur la contagion de la dothinentérie. *Arch Gén Méd* **21**: 57, 1829.
37. BOEHME D and DUBOS RJ. The effect of bacterial constituents on the resistance of mice to heterologous infection and on the activity of their reticulo-endothelial system. *J Exp Med* **107**: 523–536, 1958.
38. ELBERG SS, SCHNEIDER P and FONG J. Cross-immunity between *Brucella melitensis* and *Mycobacterium tuberculosis*. Intracellular behavior of *Brucella melitensis* in monocytes from vaccinated animals. *J Exp Med* **106**: 545–554, 1957.
39. MILLMAN I. Nonspecific resistance to tuberculosis. *Am Rev Resp Dis* **83**: 668–675, 1961.
40. DUBOS RJ and SCHAEDLER RW. Effect of cellular constituents of mycobacteria on the resistance of mice to heterologous infections. I. Protective effects. *J Exp Med* **106**: 703–717, 1957.

41. HOWARD JG, BIOZZI G, HALPERN BN, STIFFEL C and MOUTON D. The effect of *Mycobacterium tuberculosis* (BCG) infection on the resistance of mice to bacterial endotoxin and *Salmonella enteriditis* infection. *Br J Exp Pathol* **40**: 281–290, 1959.

42. MINDEN P, McCLATCHY JK, COOPER R, BARDANA EJ and FARR RS. Shared antigens between *Mycobacterium bovis* (BCG) and other bacterial species. *Science* **176**: 57–58, 1972.

43. WEISS DW. Enhanced resistance of mice to infection with *Pasteurella pestis* following vaccination with fractions of phenol-killed tubercle bacilli. *Nature (Lond)* **186**: 1060–1061, 1960.

44. WEISS DW, BONHAG RS and PARKS JA. Studies on the heterologous immunogenicity of a methanol-insoluble fraction of attenuated tubercle bacilli (BCG). I. Antimicrobial protection. *J Exp Med* **119**: 53–70, 1964.

45. LEDERER E. The mycobacterial cell wall. *Pure Appl Chem* **25**: 135–165, 1971.

46. WHITE RG. Antigens and adjuvants. *Proc R Soc Med* **61**: 1–6, 1968.

47. CROWLE AJ. Tubercle bacillary extracts immunogenic for mice. 3. Chemical degradation studies on the immunogen extracted from tubercle bacilli by trypsin digestion. *Tubercle* **43**: 178–184, 1962.

48. RIBI E, LARSON C, WICHT W and GOODE G. Effective nonliving vaccine against experimental tuberculosis in mice. *J Bacteriol* **91**: 975–983, 1966.

49. OLD LJ, CLARKE DA and BENACCERAF B. Effect of Bacillus Calmette-Guérin (BCG) infection on transplanted tumors in the mouse. *Nature (Lond)* **184**: 291–292, 1959.

50. FOLEY EJ. Antigenic properties of methylcholanthrene-induced tumors in mice of the strain of origin. *Cancer Res* **13**: 835–837, 1953.

51. PREHN RT and MAIN JM. Immunity to methylcholanthrene-induced sarcomas. *J Natl Cancer Inst* **18**: 769–778, 1957.

52. WOGLOM WH. Immunity to transplantable tumors. *Cancer Rev* **4**: 129–195, 1929.

53. KLEIN G, SJOGREN HO, KLEIN E and HELLSTROM KE. Demonstration of resistance against methylcholanthrene-induced sarcomas in the primary autochthonous host. *Cancer Res* **20**: 1561–1572, 1960.

54. KLEIN G. Tumor antigens. *Ann Rev Microbiol* **20**: 223–252, 1966.

55. WEISS DW, LAVRIN DH, DEZFULIAN M, VAAGE J and BLAIR PB. Studies on the immunology of spontaneous mammary carcinomas of mice, in: Burdette WJ (Ed), "Viruses inducing cancer." Salt Lake City, University of Utah Press, 1966, pp 138–168.

56. DEZFULIAN M, LAVRIN DH, SHEN A, BLAIR PB and WEISS DW. Immunology of spontaneous mammary carcinomas in mice. Studies on the nature of the protective antigens, in: "Carcinogenesis: a broad critique." Baltimore, Williams & Wilkins, 1967, pp 365–388.

57. WEISS DW. Immunological parameters of the host-parasite relationship in neoplasia. *Ann NY Acad Sci* **164**: 431–448, 1969.

58. WEISS DW. Immunological parameters of host-tumor relationships: Spontaneous mammary neoplasia of the inbred mouse as a model. *Cancer Res* **29**: 2368–2373, 1969.

59. VAAGE J. Non-virus-associated antigens in virus-induced mouse mammary tumors. *Cancer Res* **28**: 2477–2483, 1968.

60. VAAGE J, KALINOVSKY T and OLSON R. Antigenic differences among virus-induced mouse mammary tumors arising spontaneously in the same C3H/Crgl host. *Cancer Res* **29**: 1452–1456, 1969.

61. WEISS DW. Perspectives of host-tumor relationships. Preface and introduction, in: Weiss DW (Ed), "Immunological parameters of host-tumor relationships." New York, Academic Press, 1971, pp 1–6.

62. BENTWICH Z, WEISS DW, SULITZEANU D, KEDAR E, IZAK G, COHEN I and EYAL O. Antigenic changes on the surface of lymphocytes from patients with chronic lymphocytic leukemia (CLL). *Cancer Res* **32**: 1375–1383, 1972.

63. WEISS DW (Ed). "Immunological parameters of host-tumor relationships." New York, Academic Press, v 2 (in press).

64. WEISS DW, BONHAG RS and DEOME KB. Protective activity of fractions of tubercle bacilli against isologous tumors in mice. *Nature (Lond)* **190**: 889–891, 1961.

65. WEISS DW, BONHAG RS and LESLIE P. Studies on the heterologous immunogenicity of a methanol-insoluble fraction of attenuated tubercle bacilli (BCG). II. Protection against tumor isografts. *J Exp Med* **124**: 1039–1065, 1966.

66. ATTIA MAM and WEISS DW. Immunology of spontaneous mammary carcinomas in mice. V. Acquired tumor resistance and enhancement in strain A mice infected with mammary tumor virus. *Cancer Res* **26**: 1787–1800, 1966.

67. HELLSTROM I, HELLSTROM KE, EVANS CA, HEPPNER GH, PIERCE GE and YANG JPS. Serum mediated protection of neoplastic cells from inhibition by lymphocytes immune to their tumor specific antigens. *Proc Natl Acad Sci USA* **62**: 362–368, 1969.

68. HELLSTROM I, SJOGREN HO, WARNER G and HELLSTROM KE. Blocking of cell-mediated tumor immunity by sera from patients with growing neoplasms. *Int J Cancer* **7**: 226–237, 1971.

69. WEISS DW. Immunology of spontaneous tumors, in: Lecam L and Neyman J (Eds), "Proceedings of the Fifth Berkeley Symposium on Mathematical Statistics and Probability." Berkeley, University of California Press, 1967, pp 657–706.

70. DEOME KB, NANDI S, BERN HA, BLAIR P and PITELKA D. The preneoplastic hyperplastic alveolar nodule as the morphologic precursor of mammary cancer in mice, in: Severi L (Ed), "The morphological precursors in cancer." *Proc II Perugia Quadrennial Int Conf on Cancer,* Perugia, Division of Cancer Research, 1962, pp 349–368.

71. YASHPHE DJ and KRIPKE MC. Mammary tumors: enhancement by a nonspecific immunological stimulator and prevention of enhancement by specific immunization. *Fed Proc* **31**: 640, 1972 (Abst).

72. WEISS DW, SULITZEANU A, YOUNG L, ADELBERG M and SEGEV Y. Studies on the immunogenicity of preneoplastic and neoplastic mammary tissues of BALB/c mice free of the mammary tumor virus, in: Weiss DW (Ed), "Immunological parameters of host-tumor relationships." New York, Academic Press, 1971, pp 187–201.

73. ZBAR B, BERNSTEIN ID and RAPP HJ. Suppression of tumor growth at the site of infection with living Bacillus Calmette-Guérin. *J Natl Cancer Inst* **46**: 831–839, 1971.

74. WEISS DW. Nonspecific stimulation of the immune response by the MER fraction of tubercle bacilli. *J Natl Cancer Inst* Special Monograph Series (in press).

75. HARAN-GHERA N. Influence of host factors on leukemogenesis by the radiation leukemia virus, in: Weiss DW (Ed), "Immunological parameters of host-tumor relationships." New York, Academic Press, 1971, pp 17–25.

76. HARAN-GHERA N. Host resistance against isotransplantation of lymphomas induced by the radiation leukemia virus. *Nature (Lond)* **222**: 992–993, 1969.

77. LAPPE MA. Evidence for immunological surveillance during skin carcinogenesis. Inflammatory foci in immunologically competent mice, in: Weiss DW (Ed), "Immunological parameters of host-tumor relationships." New York, Academic Press, 1971, pp 52–65.

78. LAPPE MA. Evidence for the antigenicity of papillomas induced by 3-methylcholanthrene. *J Natl Cancer Inst* **40**: 823–846, 1968.

79. SLEMMER GL. An experimental study of premalignant mammary tissues of mice. PhD thesis, Institute for Cancer Research, Fox Chase, Philadelphia, Pa, 1971.

80. STEINKULLER CB, KRIGBAUM LG and WEISS DW. Studies on the mode of action of the heterologous immunogenicity of a methanol-insoluble fraction of attenuated tubercle bacilli (BCG). *Immunology* **16**: 255–275, 1969.
81. FILKINS JP and DI LUZIO NR. Mechanisms of gelatin inhibition of reticuloendothelial function. *Proc Soc Exp Biol Med* **122**: 177–180, 1966.
82. STERN K. Phagocytosis *in vivo* of heterologous red cells in mice with transplanted tumors. *Cancer Res* **24**: 1063–1069, 1964.
83. PASS E and YASHPHE D. Stimulation of antibody synthesis to soluble bovine gamma globulin (BGG) by a methanol-extraction residue (MER) of BCG. *Isr J Med Sci* **7**: 609–610, 1971.
84. PASS E and YASPHE D. Modulation of the immune response by a methanol-insoluble fraction of attenuated tubercle bacilli (BCG). II. Stimulation of antibody synthesis to a soluble protein, BGG. *Clin Exp Immunol* (in press).
85. WAKSMAN BH. "Atlas of experimental immunobiology and immunopathology." New Haven, Yale University Press, 1970.
86. MILLER JFAP, BASTEN A, SPRENT J and CHEERS C. Interaction between lymphocytes in immune responses. *Cell Immunol* **2**: 469–495, 1971.
87. ASOFSKY R, CANTOR H and TIGELAAR RE. Cell interactions in the graft-versus-host response, in: Amos B (Ed), "Progress in immunology." New York, Academic Press, 1971, p 369.
88. BEKIERKUNST A, LEVIJ IS, YARKONI E, VILKAS E and LEDERER E. Suppression of urethan-induced lung adenomas in mice treated with trehalose-6,6-dimycolate (cord factor) and living Bacillus Calmette-Guérin. *Science* **174**: 1240–1242, 1971.
89. SCHOENBERG MD, MUMAW VR, MOORE RD and WEISBERGER AS. Cytoplasmic interaction between macrophages and lymphocytic cells in antibody synthesis. *Science* **143**: 964–965, 1964.
90. MOSIER DE. A requirement for two cell types for antibody formation *in vitro*. *Science* **158**: 1573–1575, 1967.
91. SULITZEANU D. The affinity of antigen for white cells and its relation to the induction of antibody formation. *Bacteriol Rev* **32**: 404–424, 1968.
92. WIENER E. DNA synthesis in peritoneal mono-nuclear leucocytes. *Exp Cell Res* **45**: 450–459, 1967.
93. YASHPHE D and WEISS DW. Modulation of the immune response by a methanol extraction residue (MER) of BCG. *Isr J Med Sci* **5**: 440, 1969.
94. YASHPHE D, STEINKULLER C and WEISS DW. Modulation of immunological responsiveness by pretreatment with a methanol-insoluble fraction of killed tubercle bacilli, in: Sela M and Prywes M (Eds), "Topics in basic immunology." New York, Academic Press, 1969, pp 125–132.
95. YASHPHE DJ and WEISS DW. Modulation of the immune response by a methanol-insoluble fraction of attenuated tubercle bacilli (BCG). I. Primary and secondary responses to sheep red blood cells and T₂ phage. *Clin Exp Immunol* **7**: 269–281, 1970.
96. YASHPHE DJ. Modulation of the immune response by a methanol-insoluble fraction of attenuated tubercle bacilli (BCG). III. Relationship of antigen dose to heightened primary and secondary immune responsiveness to sheep red blood cells. *Clin Exp Immunol* (in press).
97. FRANKLIN EC. The immune globulins—their structure and function and some techniques for their isolation. *Progr Allergy* **8**: 58–148, 1964.
98. FRETER R. Agglutinating efficiency and combining capacity of Shigella and Vibrio antisera from rabbits at different stages of immunization. *J Exp Med* **105**: 623–634, 1957.
99. MOLLER G. Biologic properties of 19 S and 7 S mouse isoantibodies directed against isoantigens of the H-2 system. *J Immunol* **96**: 430–439, 1966.
100. MILES AA. The acute reactions of injury as an antimicrobial defense, in: Thomas L, Uhr JW and Grant L (Eds), "Injury, inflammation and immunity." Baltimore, Williams & Wilkins, 1964, p 162–177.

101. BURNET M. "Natural history of infectious disease." Cambridge, Cambridge University Press, 1959, pp 214–229.

102. WALFORD RL. "The immunologic theory of aging." Copenhagen, Munksgaard, 1969.

103. HELLSTROM I, HELLSTROM KE and ALLISON AC. Neonatally induced allograft tolerance may be mediated by serum-borne factors. Nature (Lond) 230: 49–50, 1971.

104. WINCHURCH R and BRAUN W. Antibody formation: premature initiation by endotoxin or synthetic polynucleotides in newborn mice. Nature (Lond) 223: 843–844, 1969.

105. BRAUN W, YAJIMA Y, JIMENEZ L and WINCHURCH RJ. Activation, stimulation and the occasional non-specificity of antibody function, in: Sterzl J and Riha I (Eds), "Developmental aspects of antibody formation and structure." New York, Academic Press, 1970, v 2, pp 799–817.

106. ARGYRIS BF. Role of macrophages in immunological maturation. J Exp Med 128: 459–467, 1968.

107. ZAALBERG OB. A simple method for detecting single antibody forming cells. Nature (Lond) 202: 1231, 1964.

108. WILSON JD. The relationship of antibody-forming cells to rosette forming cells. Immunology 21: 233, 1971.

109. GREAVES MF and MOLLER E. Studies on antigen-binding cells. I. The origin of reactive cells. Cell Immunol 1: 372–385, 1970.

110. GREAVES MF, MOLLER E and MOLLER G. Studies on antigen-binding cells. II. Relationship to antigen-sensitive cells. Cell Immunol 1: 386–395, 1970.

111. RAFF MC. Theta isoantigen as a marker of thymus derived lymphocytes in mice. Nature (Lond) 224: 378–379, 1969.

112. SCHLESINGER M. Anti-θ antibodies for detecting thymus-dependent lymphocytes in the immune response of mice to SRBC. Nature (Lond) 226: 1254–1256, 1970.

113. COHEN IR, GLOBERSON A and FELDMAN M. Stimulation of tumor growth by autosensitized spleen cells. Isr J Med Sci 7: 632–633, 1971.

114. BERRIAN JH and BRENT L. Cell-bound antibodies in transplantation immunity. Ann NY Acad Sci 73: 654–662, 1958.

115. GORER PA. Interactions between sessile and humoral antibodies in homograft reactions, in: Wolstenholme GEW and O'Connor M (Eds), "Cellular aspects of immunity—Ciba Foundation Symposium," Boston, Little, Brown and Co, 1960, pp 330–347.

116. GOWANS JL. The role of lymphocytes in the destruction of homografts. Br Med Bull 21: 106–110, 1965.

117. KLEIN E and LINDER O. Factorial analysis of the reactivity of C57Bl females against isologous male skin grafts. Transplant Bull 27: 457–459, 1961.

118. STEINKULLER C and BURTON D. Immunology of spontaneous mammary tumors in mice. Mode of action of a tumor protective fraction of tubercle bacilli (MER). Proc Am Assoc Cancer Res 7: 68, 1966.

119. KRIPKE ML and WEISS DW. Immunological parameters in the induction of murine plasma cell tumors by mineral oil, in: Severi L (Ed), "Immunity and tolerance in oncogenesis." Proc IV Perugia Quadrennial Int Conf on Cancer, Perugia, Division of Cancer Research, 1970, pp 373–391.

120. KRIPKE M and WEISS DW. Studies on the immune responses of BALB/c mice during tumor induction by mineral oil. Int J Cancer 6: 422–430, 1970.

121. BRUNNER KT, MAUEL J, CEROTTINI JC and CHAPUIS B. Quantitative assay of lytic action of immune lymphoid cells on ^{51}Cr labelled allogeneic target cells in vitro. Immunology 14: 181–196, 1968.

122. KUPERMAN O, YASHPHE D, BEN-EFRAIM S, SHARF S and WEISS DW. Nonspecific stimulation of cellular immunological responsiveness by a mycobacterial fraction. Cell Immunol 3: 277–282, 1972.

123. KUPERMAN O and WEISS DW. Further evidence for an immunological locus of action of the MER fraction of tubercle bacilli. *Isr J Med Sci* **8**: 668–669, 1972.

124. STEINITZ M and WEISS DW. Early changes in tumor cells interacting *in vitro* with sensitized lymphoid cells. *Isr J Med Sci* **8**: 666–667, 1972.

125. HERBERT WJ. Passive hemagglutination, in: Weir DM (Ed), "Handbook of experimental immunology." Philadelphia, FA Davis Co, 1967, pp 720–744.

126. YASHPHE DJ and HARAN-GHERA N. Modulation of the immune response by a methanol extraction residue of BCG: Studies on mode of action *Isr J Med Sci* **6**: 446–447, 1970.

127. SCHECHTER I. Antigenic competition between polypeptidyl determinants in normal and tolerant rabbits. *J Exp Med* **127**: 237–250, 1968.

128. TAUSSIG MJ. Studies on antigenic competition. I. Antigenic competition between the Fc and Fab fragments of rabbit IgG in mice. *Immunology* **21**: 51–60, 1971.

129. WESTPHAL O. Récentes recherches sur la chimie et la biologie des endotoxines des bactéries à Gram négatif. *Ann Inst Pasteur (Paris)* **98**: 789–813. 1960.

130. World Health Organization Technical Report Series No. 448. Factors regulating the immune response. *Int Arch Allergy Appl Immunol* **38**: 1970.

131. DRESSER DW. An assay for adjuvanticity. *Clin Exp Immunol* **3**: 877–888, 1968.

132. TANAKA A, TANAKA K, HAGIMOTO D and SUGIYAMA K. Quantitative relationship for adjuvanticity between antigen and adjuvant. *Int Arch Allergy Appl Immunol* **32**: 224–235, 1967.

133. TER-GRIGOROV VS and IRLIN IS. The stimulating effect of complete Freund's adjuvant on tumour induction by polyoma virus in mice and by Rous sarcoma virus in rats. *Int J Cancer* **3**: 760–764, 1968.

134. ASHERSON GL and ALLWOOD GG. Immunological adjuvants, in Bittar EE and Bittar N (Eds), "The biological basis of medicine." New York, Academic Press, 1969, v 4, pp 327–355.

135. BILLINGTON WD. Immunological processes in mammalian reproduction, in: Adinolfi M and Humphrey J (Eds), "Immunology and development." London, William Heinemann Medical Books, Ltd, 1969, pp 89–113.

136. FELL HB, DINGLE JT, COOMBS RRA and LACHMANN PJ. The reversible "dedifferentiation" of embryo.ic skeletal tissues in culture in response to complement-sufficient antiserum, in: Warren KB (Ed), "Differentiation and immunology." New York, Academic Press, 1968, pp 49–68.

137. GELL PGH and KELUS AS. Anti-antibodies, in: Dixon FJ Jr and Humphrey JH (Eds), "Advances in immunology." New York, Academic Press, 1967, v 6, pp 4o1–478.

138. HELLSTROM I and HELLSTROM KE. Cellular immunity and blocking antibodies to tumors. *J Reticuloendothel Soc* **10**: 131–136, 1971.

139. BRAUN W, PLESCIA OJ, RASKOVA J and WEBB D. Basic proteins and synthetic polynucleotides as modifiers of immunogenicity of syngeneic tumor cells, in: Weiss DW (Ed), "Immunological parameters of host-tumor relationships." New York, Academic Press, 1971, pp 72–82.

140. BRAUN W, LAMPEN JO, FLESCIA OJ and PUGH L. Effects of nucleic acid digests on spontaneous and implanted tumors of C3H mice, in: "Conceptual advances in immunology and oncology." *Sixteenth Ann Symp Fundam Cancer Res, 1962, Univ Texas MD Anderson Hosp Tumor Inst, Houston, Texas.* New York, Hoeber Division, Harper & Row, Publishers, Inc, 1963, pp 450–456.

SUBJECT INDEX

Anemia
  in course of infection with *Plasmodium berghei* 101–102
Antigens
  cross-reactive with streptococcal antigens 63–65
  effects of MER on clearance and body distribution of 193
Antibody-producing cells
  effects of MER on appearance of 196–203
Antimicrobial agents of microbial origin
  specificity of resistance induced by 169–173
Antiphagocytic agents, streptococcal
  host responses and 58–59

Bacteria
  host-dependent 1
Bacterial endoparasitism, *see also* Endosymbiosis
  general considerations 1–4
Bdellovibrio bacteriovorus
  as model for bacterial endoparasitism 3–11
    evolution of parasitic state 10–11
    morphological aspects 4–5
    nature of nutritional factors and conditions provided by host 8–10
    physiological aspects 5
Bovine γ-globulin
  effects of MER on responsiveness to 199–201

Cancer, animal, *see* Tumors
Cancer, development of
  cell-DNA virus interactions and 36–41
Cancer, human
  effects of MER on 188–190

Cardiohepatic toxins, streptococcal
  host responses and 56–57
Cryptococcus neoformans
  as an experimental model 133–134
  cellular response to inoculation of 140–142
  factors involved in resistance to 134
  fate of in rabbit and guinea pig 142–145
  in vitro study of 145–154
  study of host defence against
    discussion 154–159
    materials and methods 136–138
    the ring phenomenon and 134–136
    role of serum factors in ring formation 138–140

EB virus
  human lymphoma and 37–40
Endosymbiosis
  intracellular 1–2
Erythrogenic toxins, streptococcal
  host responses and 55–56

Fungi
  toxicity of 127

Hemolysins, streptococcal
  host responses and 50–52
Herpes virus
  infection by
    effect on host cell 34
    molecular aspects 29–36
  interaction with and entry of into host cell 23
  latent infection by
    molecular events 34–36
  lytic cycle of, molecular aspects 30–34
  molecular composition of 18–21

[225]